"Grace Pailthorpe was an extraordinary figure, a pioneering female surgeon, psychoanalyst and artist. The Portman Clinic, of which she is the *de jure* founder, is a unique institution that specialises in studying the roots of violent, sexual and antisocial behaviour. In some ways this parallels Surrealism's fascination with the irrational, bizarre and unconventional. This collection of Pailthorpe's writings represents a major re-appraisal of her life and her involvement with the surrealist movement."

Jessica Yakeley, *director of the Portman Clinic, consultant psychiatrist in Forensic Psychotherapy; associate medical director, clinical governance and medical director, The Tavistock and Portman NHS Foundation Trust*

"Surgeon, criminologist, psychoanalyst, surrealist, painter, Grace Pailthorpe was an intrepid pioneer in every aspect of her life, not least in her unique partnership with Reuben Mednikoff. Thanks to this indispensable collection of her theoretical writings on psychoanalysis and Surrealism, we at last have access to a remarkably original mind at work."

Elizabeth Cowling, *emeritus professor, History of Art, University of Edinburgh*

Grace Pailthorpe's Writings on Psychoanalysis and Surrealism

This book gathers the published and unpublished writings of Dr Grace Pailthorpe (1883–1971), English surgeon, specialist in psychological medicine and surrealist artist to provide an in-depth study of her work and legacy.

Pailthorpe's theoretical understanding of the psyche informed her approach to art, setting her work apart from other Surrealist artists by unifying artistic, scientific and therapeutic aims. Pailthorpe considered Surrealism to be a method of investigation into unconscious mental life and believed that it was essential that the repressed part of our minds should find expression. By bringing her artistic and theoretical work to light, Montanaro and Stefana reassert Pailthorpe's significance to the histories of both psychoanalysis and Surrealism, rendering the cross-disciplinary relevance of her work accessible to a contemporary audience.

This book will prove to be a rich resource for scholars and students interested in psychoanalysis and art history, and provides an invaluable case study for the continuing significance of visual artistic practices to clinical work.

Alberto Stefana, Ph.D., is a clinical psychologist, psychotherapist, and researcher. He has published about one hundred articles in international journals, and authored the monograph *History of Countertransference* (Routledge, 2017).

Lee Ann Montanaro, Ph.D., is a university lecturer and researcher. She specialises in twentieth century literature and art. Her research interests include Surrealism, psychoanalysis, Modernism, and comparative literature.

Grace Pailthorpe's Writings on Psychoanalysis and Surrealism

Alberto Stefana and
Lee Ann Montanaro

Routledge
Taylor & Francis Group
LONDON AND NEW YORK

Cover image: Grace Pailthorpe, Self-Portrait (n.d.), courtesy of the Dean Gallery Archive

First published 2023
by Routledge
4 Park Square, Milton Park, Abingdon, Oxon OX14 4RN

and by Routledge
605 Third Avenue, New York, NY 10158

Routledge is an imprint of the Taylor & Francis Group, an informa business

British Library Cataloguing-in-Publication Data
A catalogue record for this book is available from the British Library

Library of Congress Cataloging-in-Publication Data
Names: Pailthorpe, Grace W. (Grace Winifred), author. |
Stefana, Alberto, editor. | Montanaro, Lee Ann, 1983– editor.
Title: Grace Pailthorpe's writings on psychoanalysis and surrealism /
Alberto Stefana and Lee Ann Montanaro.
Description: Abingdon, Oxon ; New York, NY : Routledge, 2023. |
Includes bibliographical references and index. |
Identifiers: LCCN 2022027692 (print) | LCCN 2022027693 (ebook) |
ISBN 9781032366463 (hardback) | ISBN 9781032366470 (paperback) |
ISBN 9781003333098 (ebook)
Subjects: LCSH: Psychoanalysis. | Surrealism. | Psychoanalysis and art.
Classification: LCC BF173 .P225 2023 (print) |
LCC BF173 (ebook) | DDC 150.19/5–dc23/eng/20220921
LC record available at https://lccn.loc.gov/2022027692
LC ebook record available at https://lccn.loc.gov/2022027693

ISBN: 9781032366463 (hbk)
ISBN: 9781032366470 (pbk)
ISBN: 9781003333098 (ebk)

DOI: 10.4324/9781003333098

Typeset in Garamond
by Newgen Publishing UK

Contents

Figures

Foreword

This is a volume of fascinating historical documents, unfortunately long-forgotten today, but still showing an intriguing relevance to psychoanalysis and to aesthetic creativity even today. In fact, they point towards a relative neglect of that which those two disciplines have for each other. I first came across Grace Pailthorpe from a paper describing her as the first art therapist (McLagan, 1992). This is not entirely the case, and it does not entirely do justice to the work that she did from the 1930s onwards, with the British surrealist group and beyond. Instead of exploring art, Pailthorpe and her partner, Reuben Mednikoff, explored psychoanalysis as well. Not surprisingly the "couple" were a somewhat alien element of the surrealist group and hence dissociated themselves. They were intent on a new kind of psychoanalysis, not a new kind of art.

A little before Pailthorpe's immersion in psychoanalysis began in the 1920s, Freud had already studied the work of Leonardo da Vinci (Freud, 1910) and of Michelangelo (1914). But his interest was in the artistic product, the meaning of the statue of Moses to the viewer in San Pietro di Vincoli in Rome. Freud had viewed the culture daily during his stay in 1901. But Pailthorpe took a different line, not only the product but also the process.

Freud also developed his understanding of the creative *process* in dream production. And he defined that primary process with its two mechanisms, condensation and displacement. However, unconscious dream production can only be inferred at a distance in time, in the conscious waking state. Artistic production offers, potentially, a more immediate access to the creativity.

Much of Pailthorpe's more academic and professional writing (as collected in this book) is concerned with the understanding of the symbols and what they mean unconsciously as had Freud's book on his dreams (Freud, 1900). She particularly focused on birth trauma and how it is symbolised in artistic images. However, hidden within that was her slowly emerging study of the process of creating a work of art. Perhaps the birth of a person is the greatest of all creative enterprises, and possibly not so far from the birth of a piece of art. Hidden in her confident assertions in these documents is the question whether artistic creativity is intrinsic to the trauma of living. Creativity is perhaps not only the trauma of birth, but the trauma of living the next day of one's life.

I recall the exhibition of Pailthorpe's and Mednikoff's art in 2019, first at the Camden Arts Centre in London, and then subsequently at the Exchange and Newlyn Galleries in Penzance. The most arresting image was that featured as *Figure 10* in this book. There is a stunning, literally stunning, image of how the eye is assailed by what it beholds. It is the birth of an inspiration in the artist. Does it represent the trauma of the birth of that inspiration? But, it also replicates the beholder of the artistic image. Certainly, this image assaulted my eye, in Camden and in Penzance. The impact was traumatic both times. I accept that this is not quite the interpretation Pailthorpe gives her image (Chapter 3), where she is interested in the self-assault. Perhaps the significance is that the capacity to take in such a disturbing image is felt as an attack on oneself.

Much of Pailthorpe's self-analysis accomplished through her art seems to have been in reaction to her conventional analysis, with E. J. (presumably Ernest Jones). The image above may speak of a problem Pailthorpe suffered herself, but it may also speak to the process of creativity as well as the symptom of actual self-harm. There may be an aspect of the creative process in which one forms and gives birth to the image, which is experienced as the ordeal of actually birthing.

This impact of the image is not a communication in the ordinary sense of the word. It is not the same kind of "communication" as the words Pailthorpe used in writing her papers and lectures. Pailthorpe's attempt at a verbal demonstration of the self-attack of the rod through the eyeball does not capture the extreme shock of the mutilating assault. It is the image not the words that attack us. It forces itself straight into the mind without symbolisation or refined cultural manners. Such a direct impact on one's experience creates a churning in the stomach as one looks with one's eyes. It challenges the human capacity to keep our minds in order. It sprays in all directions perhaps, just as this second drawing of 1936 does. It was elaborated from a random scribble and makes a similar dismaying impact of excited incomprehension. An inscription on the back describes it as "five penises and two testicles" on a head. It is not just because of the very explicit sexual reference; the image itself, whatever one makes of it, is startling. This is an impact of a different kind. The image does the work as a direct effect leaving a scar in the mind.

These are images that convey the aesthetic experience the artist has and passes on to the viewer. But the creation begins with the immediate birth of an impression created in the artist in a moment. It is the creation of a state of mind: "We are all potential creators, having within us the divine spark that will ignite the creative flame. We are all personally interested in creation, whether we know it or not", Pailthorpe announced (Chapter 5). There is a process of several steps that goes on. It begins with the artist's creativity, initially unconsciously, and then with his talent the aesthetic object emerges, and finally there is the impact on us, the beholders. That initial step was of importance to Pailthorpe. First an "automatic" unthought-out shape, then it was elaborated into some sort of representation. That is the moment of an aesthetic elaboration building on an unconscious creation.

One could say that, perhaps without fully realising it, Pailthorpe was researching not the meanings, but the very creation of meaning itself. It is a capacity to make an unconscious impact as much as expressing a symbolic representation: "[W]hatever the act of painting may symbolise there is always an underlying reason for it. A fantasy is in progress and a story is being told" (Chapter 3). One initially gets an out-of-date feel to the rather clunky interpretation of symbols. So, it seems important to extract this element (the process of creating) in her work. Without fully realising it, she was moving on, via the surrealists, from Freud's interpreting the meaning of his own dreams in the 1890s, to her investigation of the nature of creativity.

Pailthorpe, rightly, believed the infant, being non-verbal, at the outset, must exist in a world of impressions – sound, sight, touch, etc. And so, investigating visual imagery was a more truly relevant method of psychoanalysis for accessing that early period in all our development as new-born babies. And auditory "imagery", music, is probably another prime source of those unverbalizable states of not-knowing that assault the baby. Such a non-verbal interaction is the rule before we ever speak words: "The unconscious part of one mind will speak to that of another – deep answers deep – and your response will be automatic" (Chapter 6). So Pailthorpe offered her new technique for clinical work claiming she had accessed new levels of development.

Melanie Klein too had developed a new psychoanalytic method to investigate the non-verbal periods through the analysis of children at an early age. She used toys (and drawing) for the child to express unconscious meanings and stories. As Pailthorpe said, she did not make much reference to colleagues: however she did mention one: "I am indebted to all those whose work I have previously known – and, if I may make one exception in mentioning names, I would like to say – by no means least to Melanie Klein," giving credit in the long lecture, Chapter 2. Thus, Klein too was watching the emerging aesthetic process in front of her in the very concrete terms of the play with toys. What is important is that, for Freud, dreams are analysed after their occurrence, as already formed objects with symbolic meaning. In the method of child analysis, and of Pailthorpe's artistic creations, the very moment of representing meaning in the real world, and for the gaze of others, is actually visible to the analyst. It is perhaps the case that neither Klein nor Pailthorpe had been fully aware of this new dimension they were gaining access to.

So, we should not dismiss Pailthorpe's work as simplistic intellectually-derived interpretation, rather in the manner of the "wild analysis" that Freud had condemned (Freud, 1910). The artwork points towards a newer perspective, the deeply personal impact on each other, analyst and analysand, artist and beholder, and the creation of the means of creating that impact.

In recounting the traumas and "attacks" of birth (Chapter 5), she looked forward to more contemporary issues in the psychoanalytic method. In Chapter 8, Pailthorpe conveys the way non-verbal interaction is indeed a form of "action" – screaming does not "mean" anything to mother, but it captures her attention without delay. This non-verbal interaction is important today and points to our increasing awareness of evoked feelings that are so crucial in these early stages of our lives. That "action" on another mind is the precursor of the aesthetic object that can evoke its impact on the other person.

The reader is advised to read these writings with one eye on the process of creation, on the experience of giving birth to something created, something that can create a state of mind in the other person. Pailthorpe's work straddled the significant divide between the non-verbal and verbal phases of development as does the psychoanalysis of today. Now called countertransference, and in interaction with transference, it is the acted narrative between the parties, separate from, though parallel to, the verbal communication and psychoanalytic interpretation. Psychoanalysis now attempts to give words to an understanding of something which impacts, which gives a disruption of one's experience as one looks. These writings attempt to capture that impact of an aesthetic birth. But it is a continuing theme in our lives with each other: "The whole of life has been a birth trauma repeated" (Chapter 2). To distinguish this advancing thought Pailthorpe conceived of the term "psychorealism", and she had apparently intended to devote a book-length account to it (Chapter 8). It appears she never completed it, but we now have the foundations collected by Alberto Stefana and Lee Ann Montanaro in this book.

Bob Hinshelwood
December 2021

References

Freud, S. (1900). The Interpretation of Dreams. *The Standard Edition of the Complete Psychological Works of Sigmund Freud* (*SE*) 4–5.

Freud, S. (1910). Leonardo da Vinci and a Memory of his Childhood. SE 11: 57–137.

Freud, S. (1914). The Moses of Michelangelo. *SE* 13: 209–236.

Maclagan, D. (1992). Between psychoanalysis and surrealism: The collaboration between Grace Pailthorpe and Reuben Mednikoff. *Free Associations* 1: 33–50.

Acknowledgements

Major gratitude goes to Professor Emeritus Bob Hinshelwood from the University of Essex for his help and constant support with the project. A considerable thank you is also granted to Kirstie Meehan from the Dean Gallery archive (DGA), Edinburgh, for giving immediate access to Grace Pailthorpe's diary notes and articles.

Thank you to Professor Emeritus Elizabeth Cowling from the University of Edinburgh, and Glenn Gossling from Tavistock and Portman NHS Foundation Trust for sharing their expertise, thoughts and contacts. Appreciation is also due to Reuben Mednikoff's nephew, Tony Black, and all parties who granted reproduction rights.

Credits

The authors gratefully acknowledge permission to reproduce the following material:

The analysis of a poem, G. W. Pailthorpe, *International Journal of Psychoanalysis*, (1938, 19:221–225). © Institute of Psychoanalysis reprinted by kind permission of Taylor & Francis Ltd., www.tandfonline.com on behalf of Institute of Psychoanalysis.

The scientific aspect of Surrealism. G. W. Pailthorpe, *London Bulletin* (1938–39, 7:10; 10–16). Reprinted with kind permission of Reuben Mednikoff"s nephew, Tony Black.

Primary processes of the infantile mind demonstrated through the analysis of a prose-poem, G. W. Pailthorpe, *International Journal of Psychoanalysis*, (1941, 22:44–59). © Institute of Psychoanalysis reprinted by kind permission of Taylor & Francis Ltd., www.tandfonline.com on behalf of Institute of Psychoanalysis.

Deflection of energy, as a result of birth trauma, and its bearing upon character formation, G.W. Pailthorpe, *The Psychoanalytic Review*, (1941, n. 28, pp. 305–326). Reprinted with kind permission of Guilford Press.

Transcription of speech on Surrealism for the program "Mirror for Women" (Canadian Broadcasting Corporation), G. W. Pailthorpe, (1944, July 10). Reprinted with kind permission of Darren Yearsley, Senior Media Librarian, CBC Broadcast Centre.

Chapter 1

Introduction

Grace Winifred Pailthorpe (1883–1971) was an English surgeon, specialist in psychological medicine, an associate member of the British Psychoanalytical Society (BPAS), and an artist. She was born in St Leonard's-on-Sea in Sussex on 29 July 1883, the third sibling and only girl in a family of nine brothers. Her father, Edward, was a prominent stockbroker and her mother, Anne Lavnia (nee Green), was a seamstress. Pailthorpe's family were Plymouth Brethren, and she experienced a rigidly austere puritanical upbringing against which she eventually rebelled.

Following her childhood home education due to the Plymouth Brethren practices (home-schooling would have prevented her brothers and herself from being indoctrinated by the outside world; R. Pailthorpe, 2008), Pailthorpe attended the London (Royal Free Hospital) School of Medicine for Women in the winter term of 1908–09. She received her Bachelor of Medicine and Bachelor of Surgery degrees at the University of Durham in 1914 at the age of 31. At the time, the College of Medicine consisted of 204 male students and only thirteen female students. This shows how rare it was for a woman to study medicine during that period.

After completing her medical studies, Pailthorpe went on to serve as a surgeon in the French and British Red Cross during World War I and was based in several different locations (including France, England, Malta and Italy) between 1915 and 1918. As she wrote in her war journal, her experience as a doctor for victims of the war was what led her to a lifetime practice of psychological medicine. Treating patients encouraged her to study the unconscious as she realised how sensitive and intense a patient's thoughts can become.

Once World War I came to an end, Pailthorpe decided to visit one of her brothers who lived in Australia. However, it is likely that Pailthorpe's reasons for travelling also included sightseeing and career development, which for a female doctor may not have been easy in Britain. At the time, there was very little encouragement for women to build professional careers for themselves so any female in the medical field needed to be both intelligent and strong enough to succeed in an international and largely male-dominated

DOI: 10.4324/9781003333098-1

environment. While in Australia and New Zealand, Pailthorpe worked as a general practitioner from 1919 to 1921. It is likely that it was during this period that she first became interested in criminology as, historically, criminals had often been shipped to Australia because their transportation was seen as a humane alternative to execution.

Pailthorpe's experience with victims of World War I and her work as a general practitioner encouraged her to study Freudian psychoanalysis following her return to England in February 1922. This was probably because she wanted to abandon general medicine and branch out into psychoanalysis. At that time, there was a considerable shift towards the study of mental illness. Pailthorpe sought Ernest Jones, the then president of the BPAS and editor of the *International Journal of Psychoanalysis*, because he was recognised as the first person to develop the therapeutic practice of psychoanalysis in Britain. She decided to undergo training analysis with Jones and did this from 1923 to 1930. She became an associate member of the BPAS at the start of her training. Letters from Jones to Pailthorpe, dated from 25 December 1925 to 15 November 1932, show us that Jones encouraged Pailthorpe's analytic work a lot.

Around the period that she started her training analysis, Pailthorpe also began her study of female offenders, working with and under the direction of Maurice Hamblin Smith, who is recognised as Britain's first authorised teacher of "criminology" (Garland, 2002) and the first individual to use the title of 'criminologist' (Soothill et al., 2002). Hamblin Smith believed psychoanalysis, which he saw as a "new development of psychology" (Hamblin Smith, 1922), was a way of assessing the personality of offenders and a technique for treating the mental conflicts which, he claimed, lay behind the criminal act (Soothill et al., 2002). Together, the two colleagues published a joint article entitled "Mental Tests for Delinquents, and mental conflicts as a cause of delinquency" (Hamblin Smith & Pailthorpe, 1923) in *The Lancet*. Their research article consisted of the results obtained from several mental tests which were carried out by both male and female prisoners in Birmingham Prison and concluded that mental conflict was the single cause of delinquency. The work of Hamblin Smith and Pailthorpe was the first to introduce psychoanalytic ideas to the British penal system (Cordess, 1992). Moreover, it should be noted that there were no other female criminologists working in Britain at that time and this makes Pailthorpe a pioneer in the field (Montanaro, 2010).

In 1926, upon Hamblin Smith's recommendation, Pailthorpe began her study on one hundred inmates of various Homes for girls and young women (aged between sixteen and thirty) at the request of the Central Council for Preventive and Rescue Work in London (see Pailthorpe, 1926–27). When doing her research, Pailthorpe's method involved interviews of the female prisoners as well as those who had been sent to Rescue and Preventive homes. She would spend up to ten hours in individual conversation with each inmate and make as many as six or seven visits per case (Pailthorpe, Dean Gallery archive (DGA), File 78, 20 September 1932). It became quickly evident to her that many interviewees found considerable relief and hope when they discovered she was primarily interested in how they felt about their own problems (Pailthorpe, DGA, File 78, 90, dated 1920–29) (Pailthorpe, DGA, File 78, 10 September 1932). Pailthorpe was mainly concerned with cases where she detected "mental conflict":

> As far as possible, one aimed at an outline of the life-history of the individual and her reactions to life. Her reactions to the present circumstances, her emotional mobility, her moods, the way in which she disposed of the situation in which she found herself (...) her mannerisms (...) habit spasms, tremors, blushing, sweating; (...) and her moods were all noted. Her history of states of depression and excitement was specially observed.
>
> (Pailthorpe, DGA, File 78, 39–40, dated 1920–29)

Pailthorpe's notes and conclusions on this research study attest to how her attitude toward emotions, behaviour, and somatic symptoms of those people suffering from "mental conflicts" was influenced by Freud's theory of hysteria, which was prominent in Britain in the 1920s. The originality of Pailthorpe's research resides in the focus on the causes and prevention of criminality instead of on the punishment of the criminal. On the one hand, she aimed to understand the unconscious dynamics behind violent criminal acts as well as implement psychoanalysis as a psychological treatment for offenders.

In 1932, the report for the Medical Research Council (MRC) was published. Here, Pailthorpe (1932a) claimed that for every person interviewed, it had been possible to identify an underlying psychopathological state that can and should be treated through psychotherapy and re-educational therapy. In brief, the report sought to highlight the importance of a psychological approach to the study and treatment of delinquency. However, one must bear in mind that it was subjected to much appraisal, and then subsequent forced changes, before publication (Glover, 1933; Montanaro, 2010). Meanwhile, in the same year, Pailthorpe authored a book titled *What we put in Prison* (1932b) which was not subject to "censorship" and included both clinical cases and psychoanalytically oriented theoretical considerations.

A year before the publication of the MRC report (in 1931), the Association for the Scientific Treatment of Criminals (ASTC) was established through the initiative of Edward Glover and Pailthorpe. Pailthorpe's above-mentioned report and book, which had been ready for publication since 1929, provided the backing for the endeavours of the Committee that included Ernest Jensen, Victor Neuburg, Runia Tharp, and Pailthorpe herself. The ASTC, which was renamed the Institute for the Scientific Treatment of Delinquency (ISTD) a year after its foundation, was the first British research institute dedicated to the study and treatment of criminals (Jones, 2016). In 1933 the institute opened the "Psychopathic Clinic", renamed the "Portman Clinic" in 1937, where a group of psychoanalysts, including Pailthorpe and Glover, began treating delinquent and criminal patients through psychoanalytic psychotherapy.

As part of the treatment process of the ISTD, some of the patients made drawings and paintings which, according to Pailthorpe, expressed in symbolic form the desires of their unconscious. She analysed the drawings of her patients as part of their treatment and used art as an instrument for psychological exploration, thus seeking an interactive relationship with her patient through painting. She related the forms and subjects of their art to their mental peculiarities, as their compositions often portrayed incidents and conflicts in their lives. Here Pailthorpe was using art as a therapeutic tool and her encounter, in 1935, with the commercial artist and poet Reuben Mednikoff evidently motivated her into further research of the use of art as a means of exploring the unconscious. Although Pailthorpe was intimately linked with the ISTD when it first opened and remained a vice-president until her death in 1971, any active connection ceased after meeting Mednikoff.

Mednikoff, who was familiar with psychoanalytic principles, and Pailthorpe showed an immediate interest in the other's work. They met at a party given by Pailthorpe at her house in Dorset Square in London on 21 February 1935. At the time, Pailthorpe was a surgeon and practicing psychoanalyst and Mednikoff was a commercial artist. He was 29 and she was 52. A month after their first meeting, Mednikoff introduced Pailthorpe to Surrealist automatism and encouraged her to produce her own automatic writing and drawing. After hearing his response to her interpretation of his paintings and drawings, Pailthorpe said:

> I felt that there must be somewhere a quicker way to the deeper layers of the unconscious than by the long drawn-out couch method, and I had a feeling that it was through art. At any rate it should be used in conjunction. R.M.'s quick understanding of the use and interpretation of symbols made him seem to me as probably the most suitable colleague for the research.
>
> (Pailthorpe, DGA, File 19)

These words show Pailthorpe's dissatisfaction with the classical Freudian technique (Freud, 1912, 1913, 1919) as she saw it as a misrepresentation of the demanding state of deprivation of both the analyst and the patient – to which she attributed the failure of her analysis with Jones. Pailthorpe found Klein's theory and technique (1923, 1926, 1927, 1929, 1932), with which she had probably come across through Jones or Glover, more significant and eventually made them the basis of her work.

Two months later, Pailthorpe and Mednikoff moved to a cottage in Cornwall to carry out their research. Its focus was on the psychological and therapeutic value of art which they explored in drawings, oils and watercolours. Their psychoanalytic analysis of these works was at the centre of their research project. This research went through four main phases (Maclagan, 1992): (1) from Pailthorpe and Mednikoff's first meeting until the end of their association with the British Surrealist movement (1935–40), (2) the period they spent in North America (1941–46), (3) their return to London (1946–mid-1950s), and lastly (4) the remainder of Pailthorpe's life (mid-1950s–1971). Mednikoff took on a less active role in their research once they returned to London in 1946.

Together, Pailthorpe and Mednikoff conceived what they named the "satiation-analysis" technique. In this technique, the analyst gives the patient food and drink before the analytic session to relieve any anxiety and then encourages the patient "to be as free as possible and to avoid, if he or she can, a desire to alter shapes that first appear (...) to paint without caring about results (...) to be loose and free with the paint" (Pailthorpe, DGA, File 22, C). The analyst cannot help the patient whilst painting but can make gestures of approval, permission, sympathy, and reassurance, if the patient shows any sign of needing it. Both members of the therapeutic dyad have to write notes on any feelings and thoughts they may have, and every artistic production is followed by an abundance of detailed explanations. In part, the reason for these notes is for them to be able to "go(ing) over the analytic material again and again at intervals during analysis [since it] ensures an increase in assimilation of what has come to surface before [and moreover, by doing so] each time there are added details fitted into the picture" (Pailthorpe, DGA, File 138, 1 March 1938).

Despite Pailthorpe's initial intention to make use of the conventional method in which the roles of analyst (herself) and patient (Mednikoff) were clearly delineated, the research transcended the conventional analytic boundaries and soon after they began a mutual analysis of Ferenczian (Ferenczi, 1932) flavour as there was a reversal of roles every fortnight. Their comments on their own work were part of their own self-analysis. What is striking is that Pailthorpe's interpretation of Mednikoff's art-works focused mainly on his fantasies towards her as a mother figure. Mednikoff often referred to Pailthorpe as the "mother-figure" in his notes, possibly because of the considerable age difference (she was 23 years his senior).

The spontaneous and automatic creations of Pailthorpe and Mednikoff were seen as equivalent to verbal free association in their attempt to bring the unconscious into consciousness so they could uncover the roots of the current psychopathology. Thus, in their work, the images arrived at through the free play given to the unconscious became instrumental in liberating repression. As the art historian Michel Remy (1999) says, their drawings and paintings "are the best examples of psychoanalytical examination becoming a means of liberation, based on a spontaneous outpouring of feelings, design and colour" (p. 16).

The couple clearly had a missionary faith in the therapeutic effects of such freedom which led to Pailthorpe forming a relation between unconscious wishes and infantile experiences and this eventually developed into her ideas of the "trauma of birth" (1938; see Chapter 2). Both Pailthorpe and Mednikoff investigated how anxiety at birth forms the basis of later anxieties or fears – a point of view which was originally proposed by Otto Rank (1924) "that the child's every anxiety consists of the anxiety at birth" (p. 20). Pailthorpe claimed that intrauterine ecstasy – "the pleasurable intrauterine life" or "pleasurable primal state", in Rank's words – is halted by the physical act of birth and that repressed infantile memories affect one's behaviour.

Such beliefs led Pailthorpe to produce the "Birth Trauma Series" in May 1938 as a form of therapy and to allow her to uncover the earliest preverbal anxieties and phantasies – the ones which, according to Klein (1957), are revived in the transference situation as "memories in feelings". The paintings and drawings in the "Birth Trauma Series" consist of images of pregnancy and birth. They portray the mind of the foetus during the pregnancy period. Pailthorpe maintained that the foetus is aware of every move and noise even while in the mother's womb. The "Birth Trauma Series" presents a complete picture of intrauterine and birth experiences and manifests the sensations and phantasies (which are "bound up with sensations"; Isaacs, 1952, p. 91) that a baby feels before and during birth. The series also represents Pailthorpe's attempt to explore the origins of the images of before and during birth that haunt one. There is an innate conflict between love and hate, creation and destruction, possession and the expulsion of "good" and "bad" (Klein, 1948, 1957). Pailthorpe was adamant in her belief that birth, following the infant's experience in the womb, was an epochal event which left deep impressions and shaped personalities, attitudes, and people's behaviour. She explores this idea in the "Birth Trauma Series".

Between 1938 and 1941, Pailthorpe published four articles reporting some of the results of her joint research-in-progress with Mednikoff. The first two articles emphasised how the unconscious tells its story by giving only those details that are necessary for the complete understanding of the subjects' moods, and with associations that convey the maximum effect given that every word or mark has its unconscious meaning. "The analysis of a poem" (1938; see Chapter 1) was published in the *International Journal of Psychoanalysis* (the most significant journal on psychoanalysis at the time) and "The Scientific Aspect of Surrealism" (1938–39; see Chapter 3) was published in the *London Bulletin* (the main journal outlet for Surrealist ideas in Britain). This issue of the *London Bulletin* was on sale at an exhibition of their works at the Guggenheim Jeune Gallery in Cork Street, London.

Pailthorpe refers to "The Scientific Aspect of Surrealism" in her foreword to their exhibition catalogue. Pailthorpe's article demonstrates how the couple's experiments with psychoanalysis and art were similar to the Surrealists' preoccupation with the role of the unconscious. She draws upon five of the couple's automatic drawings and paintings to support her argument and asks the audience to bear in mind that "the infantile fantasies underlying the pictures are not in consciousness at the time of painting or drawing" (Pailthorpe, 1938–39). Just as in her 1938 "birth trauma" lecture, the argument in this article is informed by Klein's school of thought as her analyses remain within the frame of Klein's theory of early infantile phantasies.

The idea expressed in these two papers was expanded on in "Primary processes of the infantile mind demonstrated through the analysis of a prose-poem" (1941a; see Chapter 4). It was published in the *International Journal of Psychoanalysis*, and in her paper, Pailthorpe describes the primary processes of the neonatal mind. Here, one should bear in mind that the prose-poems on which the analysis of two of these articles were based (i.e., Pailthorpe, 1938 and 1941a) were most likely written by Mednikoff. In the fourth article, titled "Deflection of energy, as a result of birth trauma, and its bearing upon character formation" (1941b; see Chapter 5) and published in the *Psychoanalytic Review*, Pailthorpe claims that the entire quantum of energy of an infant is regulated and controlled by the construction of defences against the repetition of pre- and particularly post-natal traumas which entail (unconscious) deviations from the life force of the subject.

In 1940, after their rupture with the Surrealist movement due to their strong reluctance to exhibit and publish only with the backing of the Surrealist group, Pailthorpe and Mednikoff left London for New York and then moved to Berkeley (Northern California) soon after. Some of their paintings and drawings were exhibited at the first exhibition of British, Canadian and American Contemporary Art which was held at the American Art Centre in early 1941. The couple's split away from the Surrealist group led Pailthorpe to rename her theory "psycho-realism" (see Chapter 8). Psychorealism and psychorealistic art were based on automatic creativeness and were the unhindered projection of psychic realities. This theory established a new understanding and conception of art, that is, the value and beauty of the symbolic value of the psyche, and the use of this symbolic language to demonstrate that the individual's emotional life is a major part of his/her whole personality which when nurtured and developed, enable the growth of the consciousness of and desire for social good. Pailthorpe's belief was that psychorealism and the technique of interpreting unconscious drawings and paintings make possible a thorough investigation into the unknown causes of social disorder and, more broadly, of every determinant and facet of human conduct. The couple were able to continue their research on the therapeutic aspect of psycho-realistic art in the USA thanks to a two-year grant they obtained from the William C. Whitney Foundation.

Following this, in the summer of 1942, Pailthorpe and Mednikoff then decided to move to Vancouver (Zemans, 1981). Pailthorpe started working at the provincial psychiatric hospital (later Riverview Hospital), and was based here until the spring of 1943 (Walsh and Wilson, 1998). The facility, which at the time was acknowledged as a model of psychiatric health care, included the Boys' Industrial School for juvenile delinquents and the Acute Psychopathic Unit. In Vancouver, Pailthorpe founded the Association for the Scientific Treatment of Delinquency (ASTD), whose objectives overlapped with those of the ISTD in London but with a specific focus on juvenile delinquency. As president of the ASTD, Pailthorpe held various lectures and spoke at conferences and round-tables. Furthermore, given that the "automatic" artistic therapy characterising the ASTD's clinical approach drew the attention of the Ladies' Auxiliary (a group of volunteer workers and art-lovers) of the Vancouver Art Gallery (the largest museum in Western Canada), in 1944, Pailthorpe was invited to give a lecture on Surrealism (Larocque, 2007).

Pailhorpe's public talk in April 1944 (see Chapter 6) was the first lecture ever given at the Vancouver Art Gallery by a surrealist artist and provided the Western Canadian mass media with the first definition of Surrealist Art as the expression of the subconscious. A second talk, where the content matched that of her first lecture, was given at the inauguration of Pailthorpe and Mednikoff's joint art exhibition (June–July 1944). The interest aroused by this exhibition in Vancouver's community was such that the Western branch of the national radio company Canadian Broadcasting Corporation asked Pailthorpe to give a brief speech (see Chapter 7) on Surrealism for the programme "Mirror for Women," in which she introduced the listeners to the history and philosophy of Surrealism and described to them the three levels of consciousness and their relationship with dreams and irrationality. By favouring the expansion of pictorial automatism within the English-Canadian media, Pailthorpe contributed to the birth of Canadian Surrealism (Larocque, 2007) and, indirectly, to the development of the psychoanalytical movement in Canada.

In March 1946 Pailthorpe and Mednikoff returned to Sussex in England, where they withdrew from the artistic scene and public life. Pailthorpe continued working both as an artist and as a clinician (a psychoanalyst in private practice and a consultant psychiatrist at the Portman Clinic), and Mednikoff became an antique dealer. Furthermore, around the first months of 1948, Mednikoff changed his name to Richard Pailthorpe, and the couple began introducing themselves as brother and sister. A few years later, in the 1950s, the couple established the first ever art therapy school in Dorking. Finally, in 1969, after more than eighteen years of retreating from the public scene, Pailthorpe exhibited some of the paintings she produced within the previous three to four years. Two years after this exhibition, Pailthorpe died due to cancer on 29 July 1971. She was eighty-eight.

What distinguishes Pailthorpe and her relationship with Mednikoff from other Surrealists was that their aims were scientific and therapeutic because they considered Surrealism to be their method of investigation into unconscious mental life. Moreover, Pailthorpe and Mednikoff's association with the Surrealists gave them the opportunity to make their research findings available to a wider audience. As her writings show, Pailthorpe specifically approached Surrealism through medicine and not art. She linked medicine with automatism yet turned to art because she believed it was important that the repressed part of our minds should find expression. Her writing shows that she was one of the few Surrealist artists who was equipped to understanding psychoanalytic theory and its relevance to art. As the reader will see in the writings collected in this book, Freud and Klein had inspired Pailthorpe's scientific understanding of the psyche, but Mednikoff and the practice of Surrealist automatism allowed her to use visual imagery from the subconscious mind to create art.

Nevertheless, although Pailthorpe is currently recognised by art historians as a significant British surrealist painter of the 20th century (Maclagan, 1998; Rosemont, 1998; Wilson, 1998; Remy, 1999), since she was initially a relatively obscure figure whose work was barely recognised by her peers, she was and still is scarcely acknowledged by psychoanalysts and historians of psychoanalysis. Indeed, when searching for "Pailthorpe" in the Psychoanalytic Electronic Publishing (PEP) Archive (Date of access: August 30, 2021) there are only seventeen articles (eight prior to and nine following her death) that

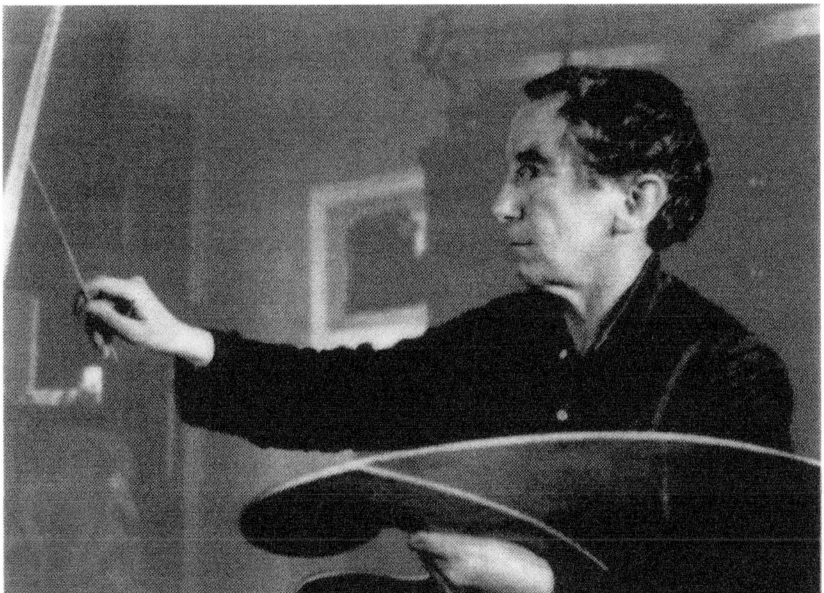

Figure 1.1 Grace Pailthorpe (1883–1971).

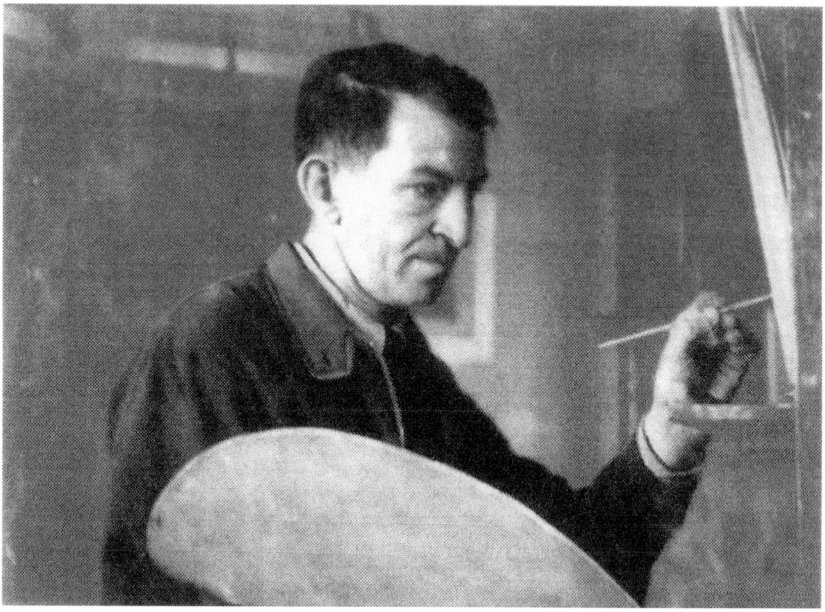

Figure 1.2 Reuben Mednikoff (1906–1972).

include her name, four of these (Brierley, 1933; Glover, 1933; Fenichel, 1939; Thomas, 1943) are short article/book reviews or summaries, three are by one of the editors of the present book (Stefana, 2018a, 2018b, 2019), and only one (Maclagan, 1992) is an in-depth study of her work. Pailthorpe's work with Mednikoff is one of the few examples of an artist and his painting playing an active role in a psychoanalytic context as their images call for a psychological response. Yet, despite its historical value, Pailthorpe's theoretical work is not fully recognised. Hence, the purpose behind this collection of her writings is to present them to the public domain.

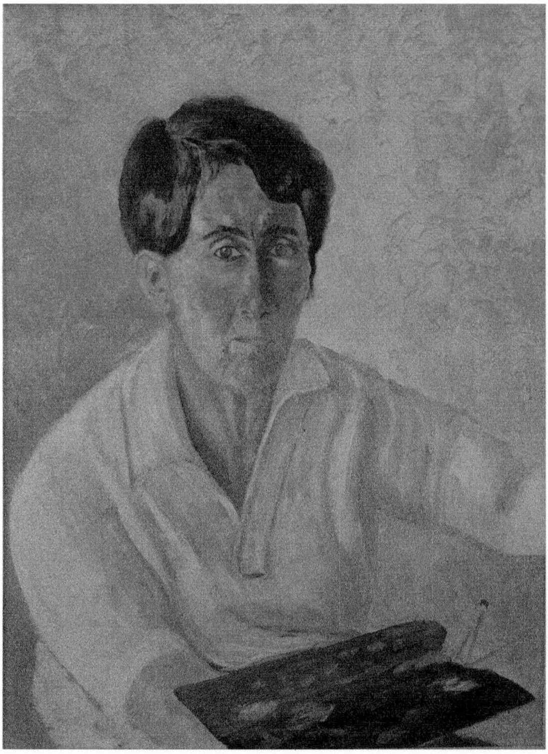

Figure 1.3 Grace Pailthorpe, self-portrait owned by Bob Hinshelwood.

References

Brierley, M. (1933). General: Anon. Psychology of delinquency. *British Medical Journal*, October 29th, 1932, p. 801. *International Journal of Psycho-Analysis* 14: 109.

Cordess, C. (1992). Pioneers in forensic psychiatry. Edward Glover (1888–1972): Psychoanalysis and crime – A fragile legacy. *Journal of Forensic Psychiatry & Psychology* 3: 509–530.

Dean Gallery Archives (DGA), Edinburgh. Accessible at www.dswebhosting.info/NGS/CalmViewA/TreeBrowse.aspx?src=CalmView.Catalog&field=RefNo&key=GMA+A62

Fenichel, O. (1939). PAILTHORPE, GRACE W.: The Analysis of a Poem. Int. Journal of PsA., XIX/2. *Internationale Zeitschrift für Psychoanalyse* 24: 352.

Ferenczi, S. (1932). *The clinical diary of Sándor Ferenczi*. Harvard University Press, 1988.

Freud, S. (1912). Recommendations to physicians practising psycho-analysis. *The standard edition of the complete psychological works of Sigmund Freud* (*SE*) 12, pp. 109–120.

Freud, S. (1913). On beginning the treatment (Further recommendations on the technique of psychoanalysis I). *SE* 12, pp. 121–144.

Freud, S. (1919). Lines of advance in psycho-analytic therapy. *SE* 17, pp. 159–168.

Garland, D. (2002). Of Crimes and Criminals: The Development of Criminology in Britain. In: M. Maguire, R. Morgan, & R. Reiner (Eds.), *The Oxford Handbook of Criminology*, Third Edition, Oxford University Press.

Glover, E. (1933). What We Put in Prison: By G. W. Pailthorpe, M.D. (Williams & Norgate, London, 1932. Pp. 159. Price 5 s. net.). *International Journal of Psycho-Analysis* 14: 278–279.

Hamblin Smith, M. (1922). *The psychology of the criminal*. Methuen.

Hamblin Smith, M., & Pailthorpe, G. W. (1923). Mental tests for delinquents, and mental conflict as a cause of delinquency. *Lancet* 2: 112–114.

Isaacs, S. (1948). The nature and function of phantasy. *International Journal of Psycho-Analysis*, 29, 73–97.

Jones, D. W. (2016). *Disordered personalities and crime*. Routledge.

Klein, M. (1923). The development of a child. *International Journal of Psycho-Analysis* 4: 419–474.

Klein, M. (1926). Infant analysis. *International Journal of Psycho-Analysis* 7: 31–63.

Klein, M. (1927). Symposium on child-analysis. *International Journal of Psycho-Analysis* 8: 339–370.

Klein, M. (1929). Personification in the play of children. *International Journal of Psycho-Analysis* 10: 193–204.

Klein, M. (1932). *The psycho-analysis of children*. Hogarth Press.

Klein, M. (1948). A contribution to the theory of anxiety and guilt. *International Journal of Psychoanalysis* 29: 114–123.

Klein, M. (1957). Envy and gratitude. In: *Envy and gratitude and other works. 1946–1963*. Hogarth Press.

Larocque, Y. M. (2007). Grace Pailthorpe et Reuben Mednikoff à Vancouver. La transmission du surréalisme au Canada anglais, 1942-1946. *RACAR: revue d'art canadienne / Canadian Art Review* 32: 35–44.

Maclagan, D. (1992). Between psychoanalysis and surrealism: The collaboration between Grace Pailthorpe and Reuben Mednikoff. *Free Associations* 1: 33–50.

Maclagan, D. (1998). Making for mother. In: N. Walsh, & A. Wilson (Eds.) *Sluice Gates of The Mind: The Collaborative Work of Pailthorpe and Mednikoff*. City Art Gallery.

Montanaro, L. A. (2010). *Surrealism and psychoanalysis in the work of Grace Pailthorpe and Reuben Mednikoff, 1935–1940*. Doctoral dissertation, University of Edinburgh.

Pailthorpe, G. W. (1926–27). Report on a psychological investigation of the inmates of preventive & rescue homes in London. Dean Gallery Archives, (GMA A62/1/007). Accessible at www.dswebhosting.info/NGS/CalmViewA/TreeBrowse.aspx?src=CalmView.Catalog&field=RefNo&key=GMA+A62

Pailthorpe, G. W. (1932a). *Studies in the psychology of delinquency*. Medical Research Council.

Pailthorpe, G. W. (1932b). *What we put in prison and in preventative and rescue homes*. Williams and Norgate.

Pailthorpe, G. W. (1938). The analysis of a poem. *International Journal of Psycho-Analysis* 19: 221–225.

Pailthorpe, G. W. (1938–39). The scientific aspect of Surrealism. *London Bulletin* 7: 10–16.

Pailthorpe, G. W. (1941a). Primary processes of the infantile mind demonstrated through the analysis of a prose-poem. *International Journal of Psycho-Analysis* 22: 44–59.

Pailthorpe, G. W. (1941b). Deflection of energy, as a result of birth trauma, and its bearing upon character formation. *Psychoanalytic Review* 28: 305–326.

Pailthorpe, G. W. (1944). Transcription of speech on Surrealism for the program "Mirror for Women" (Canadian Broadcasting Corporation). July 10.

Pailthorpe, R. (2008). Personal communication with Lee Ann Montanaro.

Rank, O. (1924). *The trauma of birth*. Routledge, 1999.

Remy, M. (1999). *Surrealism in Britain*. Ashgate Publishing Company.

Rosemont, P. (1998). *Surrealist women: An international anthology*. University of Texas Press.

Soothill, K., Peelo, M., & Taylor, C. (2002). *Making sense of criminology*. Polity.

Stefana, A. (2018a). Die Rolle der ästhetischen Erfahrung im künstlerischen Schaffensprozess nach Marion Milner. *Psyche - Zeitschrift für Psychoanalyse* 72:50–71.

Stefana, A. (2018b). From *die Traumdeutung* to the squiggle game: A brief history of an evolution. *American Journal of Psychoanalysis* 78:182–194.

Stefana, A. (2019). Revisiting Marion Milner's work on creativity and art. *International Journal of Psychoanalysis* 100:128–147.

Thomas, G. (1943). Deflection of Energy, as a Result of Birth Trauma, and its Bearing Upon Character Formation: Grace W. Pailthorpe. Psa. Rev., XXVIII, 1941, pp. 305–326. *Psychoanalytic Quarterly* 12: 593–593.

Walsh, N., & Wilson, A. editors (1998). *Sluice gates of the mind: The collaborative work of Pailthorpe and Mednikoff*. City Art Gallery.

Wilson, S. (1998). *Surrealism painting*. Phaidon Press.

Zemans, J. (1981). Jock Macdonald: *The inner landscape: A retrospective exhibition*. Art Gallery of Toronto.

Chapter 2

The analysis of a poem[1]

The following poem, which was accepted for publication in one of the leading literary magazines, was written during the writer's analysis.

KAROO

What ails me now?
What ails this land—bare, barren of all green life? … fretted by hot
winds, hot curling puffs? … and all is still again—hard, granite
rock.
And I?
I wander listlessly from rock to rock,
searching to find one flicker of life within its hidden creases.
But hope dies.
Nothing is found but molten metal—the dung of a thousand sun-strained
mornings.
The sun, sullen in its powerful might, stares brazenly on Earth's
blackened
loins
and, staring, stabs relentlessly at dugs it has sucked dry.
My life is stilled at last—scorched.
Wrenched from the burnt-up corpse, the spirit rises in fast gyrations …
mounts into the face of the sullen monster
and strikes, with all life's force, its callous, brutal disc:
in the striking is released in a myriad scattered echoes:
in this last act ascends, descends—everlastingly—
in immortal waves.

The objective in presenting the analysis of this poem is to exemplify the extent to which the unconscious mind works in the creation of poetic literature. The style of it is in the modern vogue of 'vers libre'. Rhyming is absent. Rhythm is abundantly present and adapted throughout to the feeling-tone of the subject matter.

DOI: 10.4324/9781003333098-2

The poem was written by the patient during a spell of analysis. This occurred in the lavatory while making a constipated stool. When writing, he was aware that his constipation was in some way connected with the poem. Recently, analysis had been bringing into consciousness the period in the patient's history when bottles were being exchanged for milk from a mug and more solid food; and the replacement of the bottle-teat by a dummy-teat. It is well-known that change of food usually brings about a temporary constipation, or its opposite—diarrhoea. This, of course, may be so slight as to pass notice; but, generally speaking, this statement holds true.

Analysis of the poem at the time of writing gave the following interpretation of the unconscious material which was being dramatized.

> The sun, sullen in its powerful might …

This was felt to relate to the mother's or nurse's stern demand for the morning stool to be made.

> Dugs it has sucked dry.

This referred to a dummy-teat in place of a bottle.

the dung of a thousand sun-strained mornings.

The sun's dung is the mother's dung. And the sun's dung and the child's dung are one and the same for all dung belongs to the mother. This had been made abundantly clear from previous analysis. In the case of this patient, up to this point in analysis, the sun, contrary to the usual unconscious meaning or symbolization given to it, represented the mother almost entirely. Later it was also used as a father symbol. This was all that was brought forward in the interpretation of the unconscious meanings of the poem at the time of its creation.

Six months later, the patient was typing the poem and suddenly became aware that every word had its unconscious meaning; and, at the same time, saw in a mental vision the early episode that was the activating stimulus of its creation. I give his own words:

> While transcribing my poem I was interested to see how clear it was to me now. I found myself typing it with a running commentary going on in my head and seeing the whole scene of its origin. … I see myself sitting on my chamber, a child of one year or thereabouts. I have struggled ineffectively to produce my morning stool. Nurse stands over me, angry and demanding.
>
> "What ails me now?" is myself wondering why nothing comes. "*What ails this land*"—translated, is "What is the matter with my insides?" "*bare, barren of all green life*" is referring to the absence of babies (green life) from my stools. (The expectation of finding babies in the stool was already a conscious realization to the patient.)
>
> "Fretted by hot winds, hot curling puffs, and all is still again" indicates two things. Firstly, colly-wobbles or flatus and, secondly, the heat of my face produced with and by each terrific effort at expelling my stool.

"All is still again" refers to the rest taken after such an effort. "*And I? I wander listlessly from rock to rock*" shows a lessening of effort. I am tired now, but am still hoping that something will happen and the reluctant stool will emerge for I am still searching to find "*one flicker of life within its hidden creases*"—the creases of "*granite rock*" of constipated fæcal matter which is pressing on my anus but cannot be moved.

The tiny "fart" that always, when it comes, helps on a constipated stool is the "one flicker of life" which is being searched for. With the absence of this "*hope dies*". Nothing is found but "*molten metal*", the end-result of "*a thousand sun-strained mornings*". This refers to the many mornings on which I have had to suffer the anger of the waiting nurse and the consequent constipation. The nurse is there, standing over me, demanding my stool, hurrying me over my stool and pouring down on my defenceless head her hot anger at my delays; and thus, through the fear engendered, drying up my stool inside. (Analysis has shown constipation as well as diarrhoea to be the result of fear among other things.)

"The sun, sullen in its powerful might, stares brazenly on Earth's blackened loins"—the nurse stands sullenly by and stares menacingly at me. My loins are "*blackened*"—this is a reference to the blackness that invades one's eyes and, therefore, one's whole being when a long, terrific and sustained effort is made to expel the stool while holding the breath.

"And, staring, stabs relentlessly at dugs it has sucked dry" refers to my childish belief that the nurse is depriving me of valuable food-milk by her matutinal demands and has thus dried up the contents of my bowel; for, if it were not so, there would be the usual flow of "er-er". ("Er-er" was the patient's baby-word for stools. Previous analysis had shown this episodic constipation to have occurred at the moment of weaning from bottles and, at the same time, when solid food was being introduced into the daily diet.)

"My life is stilled at last" means I am exhausted and cannot make any further effort.

"Scorched. Wrenched from the burnt-up corpse ..."—the corpse is the "er-er" baby that I feel is dead within me, for it does not move to come out in the usual way. The expectation of a baby out of my stools was frequently present.

The rest of the poem is a picture of the hate roused in me at this bafflement to my life's expression. She, "the sullen monster", is the cause of this death to me and my "er-er" baby. Into her face I fly and strike myself to pieces on her "*callous, brutal disc*". Life is poured out in hate and, in so doing, finds life again—"*in this last act ascends, descends—everlastingly—in immortal waves*".

The idea of ceasing to exist is impossible of comprehension to the unconscious. The freedom that is desired is freedom from the cause of the '*stilled life*' within; that is, from the stoppage of the peristaltic wave or rhythm. The idea of the part as the whole is evident here—the microcosm as the macrocosm. Each piece of the many pieces of the broken entity flung wide from the impact with the sun's '*callous, brutal disc*' lives separately and entirely as a whole throughout eternity. Immortality is held untouchable. Death to gain immortal freedom—to escape the frustration that is killing the life within. 'Flying to death to escape death'—a favourite expression of the patient's—is once more used as a means of avoiding the otherwise inescapable. Previously the phrase 'Flying to death to escape death' had been used in relation to an unknown fear, later seen through analysis to be the fear of punishment. This was one aspect of it. Here, in the subject under review, is another—that anything that threatens life can only be avoided by taking the way of death. Death in either case is a gaining of release from intolerable tension. The gain of life through death was connected with the Christ myth—'Except ye die and be born again ye cannot enter the kingdom of heaven' (that is, enter life). This phrase was frequently on the lips of the patient. Fear or block to expression, that is the act of living, are two major reasons, amongst others, for suicide. The writer of this poem had been very near death for these reasons on at least two occasions.

The peculiar interest of this poem lies in the fact that every single phrase had its unconscious reason. The unconscious inspired the poem. Not a single phrase or word was superfluous to the story it had to tell. Equally remarkable is the extraordinary way in which the unconscious selects from reality-experience the subject-equivalents to suit the unconscious needs. Its power of selection reaches an exactitude that is almost mathematic in its accuracy of sensation equivalents, for the unconscious situation is perfect in its association to the Karoo. The unconscious seizes any material available to hand to stage its story. The opportunity was here since the patient had seen the Karoo: and the dried, burnt-up land and fiery sun lent itself so aptly as 'props' to the dramatization of this episode.

While the poem was being written there was no mental consciousness of the Karoo. There was merely the feeling on the part of the patient that it was all due to his constipation at the time.

Note

1 This analysis was first published in the *International Journal of Psycho-Analysis* (1938, 19:221–225).

Chapter 3

The Birth Trauma Lecture (1938)

Lecture on drawings. Being an extract from a research now in its final stages[1]

Before I begin this lecture, I want to say that it is a demonstration of analytic material only. I cannot, for want of space and time, make reference to others' work in relation to the unconscious and Art, nor am I fully qualified since, of necessity, for the period of the research I have not kept up with analytic literature. I am indebted to all those whose work I have previously known – and, if I may make one exception in mentioning names, I would like to say – by no means least to Melanie Klein.

My reasons for inviting you to listen to the demonstration I shall give this evening are manifold.

As we know, "time waits for no man". In such a period of instability and upheaval as we are experiencing today the world is looking towards psychology as its last hope in a "lost cause". Anything, therefore, that can add to our knowledge of mental functioning: that can ensure therapeutic results in psycho-analysis: that can hasten the process of securing these therapeutic results must certainly be given to the scientific world as soon as it can possibly be done.

I have been engaged in a research over a period of four years. I claim, as a result of this work, to have found a method by which psychoanalysis can be shortened and yet is more thorough in its exploration of the unconscious than has been hitherto possible. Further, it is a method which, I am of the opinion, must inevitably bring about therapeutic results, where organic lesion is not present.

My difficulty has been whether, in view of the fact that I have actual proof of my claims, I should wait until I have set out the vast amount of detail amassed in perfect order or give it to you now as it is. If I wait till it is completed, as I must do if I remain without financial help, it will take me another two years to complete it. If I have the necessary help, I shall be able to have it, or some part of it, ready in six months.

It is for this reason I have abstracted a short section of an analysis for demonstration purposes. Just as what I show you today is full of information and detail, so too is every part of the analysis of this subject. In the final

DOI: 10.4324/9781003333098-3

presentation I am proposing to make in book form there will be the complete analyses, by this method, of two individuals; namely, myself and my colleague R. Mednikoff. As Haldane would put it, we have been our own rabbits in the research.

In the book I shall also give excerpts from the analyses of other of my patients who have experienced the same treatment.

If I should excite your interest this evening, I shall have definite proposal to make.

With others, I have dissatisfied for a long time with the results of psycho-analysis; and, when certain ideas crystallised out in my mind, as a result of definite psychological experiences I came across both in myself and in my patients, I set to work to put them to the test. The results have been abundant beyond all expectation. I cannot enumerate them here, nor is there time to demonstrate all the results in one short session, but I can say that what I am giving you as a sample of the research material is true in quality of all the research material.

I hope to demonstrate with what extraordinary detail and accuracy the unconscious can be persuaded to "speak".

Paintings and drawings come into this analysis, but they are not essential material in analyses by the method adopted in this research. I have chosen to extract a section which includes drawings as an example for demonstration since it serves a double purpose. Not only does it show in the minutest detail the working of mind, from the earliest possible moment, but it throws a very considerable light on the function of Art. It unfolds in detail what is already known in theory, viz. the work of the unconscious in the realm of Art. There will not be time, however, to amplify this in this paper.

Before I proceed to the demonstration itself, I want to say that I shall not be able to say anything about the method adopted to get these results. This will be recorded in the right place.

The rapidity of the method in obtaining results and the thoroughness of it is manifest in what you will hear and see today.

I have chosen as an example to present to you a fraction of my own analysis. I could have given you just as easily a section from the analysis of my colleague, but I have chosen to present my own case for several reasons. These will become obvious before the finish.

The period of time expended upon the portion of analysis I shall present was twelve days. This was broken in the beginning by a seven-day visit to London.

I begin with the end of a previous eruption of unconscious material and its clarification, thus showing how one part led to the next. Then follows a complete picture of birth experiences. It will demonstrate that not only is all experience recorded, but that mind is active and at work even at the time of birth. It will show how at this early date the mind of the infant sought for a reason to explain to itself the transition from the comfort of a quiescent womb to the turbulence and menacing experiences of the processes of being born and those immediately following birth. It will show some of the effects of these events on the subject's subsequent life and development.

Previous to the emergence of the birth trauma into consciousness, an episode that had occurred at the age of three days, had appeared and the fears in relation to it had been resolved. It appeared that I had been fed; but continued, in spite of this, to have a hunger-pain. This was due to indigestion and a vomiting attack. Later, when asleep, I had dreamt that I had eaten the breast and that it was inside me: and that by this device I should never again be hungry. When the time came for the next bottle-feed, the teat, and possibly the rate at which the milk came, caused me to choke to the point of blacking-out, that is, becoming unconscious. This was registered by my infant-mind as an attack on me because I had eaten the breast. This revelation was followed by the recognition of the reasons for many aspects of my reactions to life. As I have an already too long lecture ahead of me I do not propose to enumerate these realisations now but to run through the drawings which ended that phase of analysis and then to pass on to what followed in subsequent analysis. The realisation that the choke was not due to reprisal for my eating the breast made the next piece of analysis possible. In brief: by understanding what immediately preceded the emergence of the birth trauma into consciousness you will be able to appreciate the movement and tempo of the entangled unconscious towards the freedom of consciousness.

I will now show you the drawings of this series and will give you the notes which were made after the drawings were finished. It is important to hold this in mind.

Slang or baby words are used as they came into my mind or were written at the time.

I started this drawing by trying to put myself into the womb again (top left) but crossed it out and then did other scribbles. I felt that the large shape on the extreme right was me dancing or throwing myself about; partly in excitement and partly as a stretch.

The left figure is me. I am definitely kicking about this time and am full of milk (yellow). The figure on the right is me – empty of milk, thin and emaciated – saying to myself, "I may get full of milk and kick with excitement now". The red lock of hair also feels to me to be an extra mouth.

I was not feeling too good and had a feeling of indigestion while drawing. In this painting I am lying cuddled up on a blue shawl, on a lap. The red thing on my back is a warm hand. I think it has a double meaning – being also placenta. I felt that the black background was as much womb as dress. (Black was worn by nurses or mothers when I was a baby). I think this painting is saying,

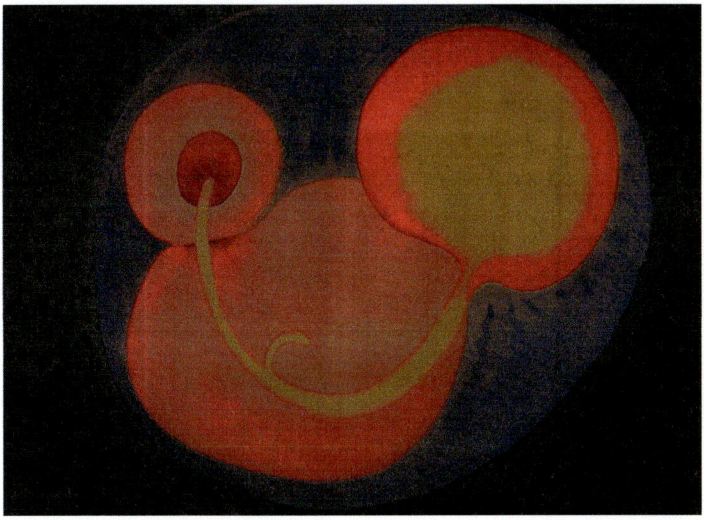

Figure 3.1 Birth Trauma Series 2: May 3, 1938, No. 3.

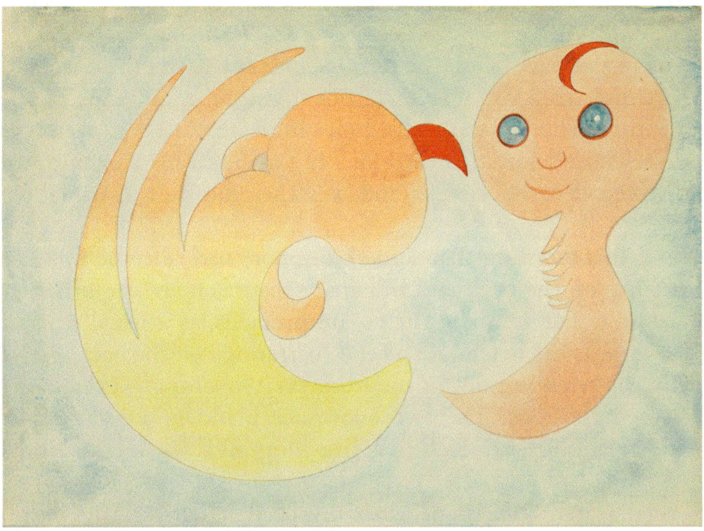

Figure 3.2 Birth Trauma Series 3: May 4, 1938, No. 6.

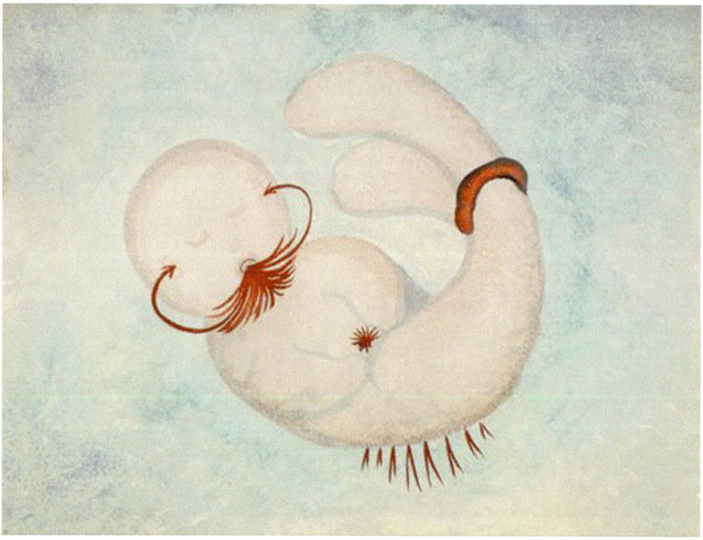

Figure 3.3 Birth Trauma Series 5: May 6, 1938, No. 5.

"I wish they would put something hot on my back like I had on me inside", (that is, inside the womb).

Here I am in a lap again. A hand (the red shape) is smacking my back and forcing up everything from my inside – from my mouth and anus as the two arrows pointing to the two dark blue holes indicate. As I was drawing, I had begun to belch and found myself sucking again. This smacking of my back must have been too violent and was therefore felt as attack or punishment.

I felt on waking this morning that something more had to come up. The belching, the patting on the back and the final exhaustion are the bits that had to be isolated or, rather, itemised (by my unconscious, as it usually does). Here, in this drawing, is the belching and the "battering" on the back.

Here everything is trickling out of me from every opening – eyes, nose, mouth and between the legs. The two enormous bladders are my arms. This, I feel, merely symbolise the feeling of big-lumpiness when one's limbs go dead.

Here is the final state. This is me with my head fallen forward, dead. Black = dead. My neck is pulled long by my lolling head. The unconscious demanded the word "FINIS", so I put it in. I began yawning after this in a way that is usually the sign of the conclusion of a bit of analytic work. To make sure that this was the finish I did one more drawing.

This merely repeated the final episode of exhaustion resulting in a black-out. The drawing indicates that I feel just a limp head (the black dot) on a

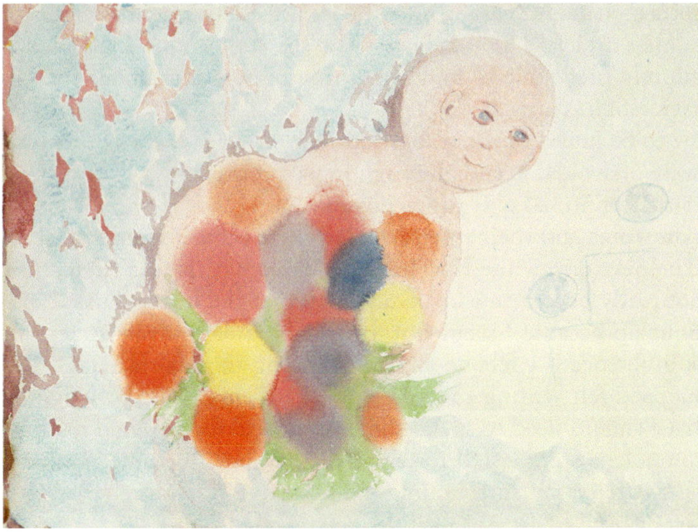

Figure 3.4 Birth Trauma Series 6: May 11, 1938, No. 1.

long neck (the thin line). The head comes off = blacks-out. The small figures at bottom right illustrate the process of the final fading away to nothing, to the black-out.

The notes continue.

Yet although the unconscious had definitely said "finis", there may be more to come as I don't reel exactly free. I don't feel anything. Probably I am too exhausted to feel anything yet or there may be something more to come.

Belching is now coming freely since this morning.

With regard to being pommelled on the back when choking: I have always been afraid of that being done to me while I am in a choke. It always seems to me a last straw – some extra pain and discomfort to be coped with when already one is dying from the choking. I must have felt too that it was, in part, a hitting of things out of me, viz. the things which I had eaten in fantasy or dream, as, for example, the breast.

The blacking-out is the final attack – a stretching of a neck and the pulling a head off.

The unconscious is most imperative that every detail shall be given and understood. My unconscious can only realise one thing at a time: first, that I was not being made to vomit because I was aggressive towards the nipple and breast; second, that pommelling the back was not a punishment; third, that the exhaustion and blacking-out (becoming unconscious) was not a punishment. Each of these three realisations emerged separately, but in the sequence given.

Reasonless attack cannot be tolerated by a baby completely dependent and helpless in another's hands. Reasons must be found. Punishment is easier to bear than reasonless attack. This I believe to be the real origin of the idea of guilt. It is infinitely preferable to find something to be guilty about than to be subjected to reasonless attack.

Relief is now to be found in the realisation that "attacks" were not reasonless fury but were unavoidable and although in part mistakenly, were applied to relieve the situation in so far as it was possible.

After these drawings and their interpretation there came a week's break in the analysis. The next day, while travelling to London in the car I remarked that I could not really become aware of anything that the last few days' analysis had brought up because I seemed to be in a kind of far-away state. But there was this difference – I felt no anxiety in being in that state, as I had previously done, and felt willing to let things take their course. I thought it was natural that I should need to spend some time "soaking up" and resting.

The semi-somnolent state lasted for three days before I became normally alert again and aware of my surroundings in an active way rather than as a passive onlooker at life.

The visit to London on this occasion was more like a holiday than previous visits had been. The time was less cluttered up with appointments. There was time for leisure and pleasure.

The whole morning following the return from London was spent in drawing. The previous night I had a dream which I had recounted to R.M. (Mednikoff) and then set aside for future consideration.

The notes on the morning's drawings were as follows:

> The outer orange oval is the mummy-womb. The orange outline within this is me. The top oval part of this is my head which is looking into the womb. The picture my eye sees when looking into the womb is drawn in the eye itself (the central brightly coloured disc). The orange centre to this multi-coloured eye is again myself and at each end I have a mouth which is being fed by a breast-nipple. All the pink shapes in this eye are breasts: the yellow indicates abundance of milk: the blue, green and red are the other things that are comforting in a womb – red = warmth, blue = water and the comfort of being cushioned, and green, I think, is body odour. As I was doing this drawing my unconscious said, "that is why you are fond of the kaleidoscope. You saw all these colours while in the womb".

It is true that when shutting one's eyes in darkness a number of colours can often be seen, but that does not seem to be what my unconscious meant. I think what it meant was that the feelings of pleasure I derived from the perfect balance in movement, the rhythmic waves in pulsation and the complete comfort of food from the mother-blood were akin to the vibrations associated with the colours mentioned; that they gave a pleasure akin to these intra-uterine comforts.

Summing up: the story of this picture is that I am looking into the mother-womb and seeing myself in the womb enjoying all these comfort-sensations.

The blue shape is the womb and the central pale pink disc with the darker pink disc in it is my head with a mouth. The larger dark pink shape below this is my body. The yellow horse-shoe shape extending from a yellow disc below my body to my mouth is a nipple feeding me from a mother-breast. The other objects are milk (yellow), blood (brown) and faecal matter (green).

This picture seems a duplicate of the last but with this difference – that I am now *in* the womb and not merely looking into it.

Here I, the pink object on the left, am definitely and safely ensconced within the womb (blue). The dark surround, which is rhythmical and vibrating, is comforting because of its darkness. The pink body and head of myself is undifferentiated except for one feature: the mouth. Into the mouth is going the yellow teat. The red and yellow shape to the right is a composite of the placenta and breast. The little yellow branch coming off the elongated nipple is equally the umbilical cord. I think this painting is saying, "I wish the placenta-breast that fed me through my belly while inside mother would now feed me, inside mother, through my mouth". It is interesting to note the directness of the unconscious in making a statement and its economy of language, for again the mouth is the only feature depicted.

This is another womb picture and is showing the sensation I have from the mother-blood being pumped into me. I feel this at every point as indicated by the faint, rhythmic, purple marks on my body: not only inside the body but impinging upon my outer surface all round, as shown by the purple and pink blobs around my head.

In this the same idea is present but it is conveying more warmth by the colour and I think the unconscious demanded this painting merely to add, or emphasise, the pleasure in the general feeling of warmth and vibration; that is, the gentle titillation of my whole body.

This is repetitive in a sense, but I feel that what the picture is saying is that when all these various rhythms are playing on my body, and inside it, that my body itself is aglow with light and every colour.

I feel these drawings are the explanation to the kaleidoscope reference in the notes on No. 1 of this series. That somehow all that impinges upon and within the growing embryo is comparable in its effect on the senses to all the colour vibrations of the spectrum. If this be so it means that there is a bio-logic importance in every variety of vibration felt by the embryo or foetus in addition to the importance of the actual physical matter (from the mother) given to form life.

We will now return to the dream mentioned as having preceded this series of drawings.

Before reading you the notes on the dream I would like to say that this dream was the response of the unconscious to the holiday it had had from analysis. The rest from the shock of the previous realisation is complete: the unconscious is ready to continue its work. The dream is a direct and immediate bringing up of the unconscious material – as if the unconscious were saying, "This is what I want to know all about next". Here is the dream.

When I woke this morning, I was conscious of having dreamt analytically and that the vague content of the dream was that I wanted to go inside the womb to eat but that I would be attacked if I did. The final bit of the dream had to do with a car in which, I think, I was. But this part is vague as I seem also to see the car as an onlooker would. The car suddenly starts turning over on its side and tipping out everyone inside it. It then rights itself and stays still. It does not appear to be much damaged although the wheels on the near side were very wobbly looking.

In view of the drawings which I did following this dream, it seems as if this is a re-experience of birth. Before I was fully awake, I dreamt I struggled to tell R.M. some of what I could hold of the dream and I said to him, "If one eats things inside mother one is attacked" (=punished). Thus, I am saying in the dream, "I would like to go back to the womb and feed inside mother but if I do, I will be attacked".

During the first drawing of this morning, I now recollect thinking, "what is there to attack me in the womb?" and wondered if "I should draw in other babies"; but my unconscious would not have this. It seems now, in interpreting the dream, that what I expect as an attack or punishment if I should get back into the womb would be the repetition of the birth process – "being turned out of the motor-car" (=womb and mother). That is what was felt to be the first punishment of all.

About the very end of the last bout of analysis and just before going to London the words "three days" had been coming up in my mind and I had once mentioned it to my colleague as possibly meaning three breast-feeds. It is quite clear from what has followed that it must have been within a very short time of my birth. The word "Finis", on the final drawing, was, as far as my unconscious was concerned, a definite statement. From that moment and for the next few days I was quiescent, withdrawn, with a far-away-feeling and with nothing active going on in my mind. I was once again in the womb. It seemed to me as if I were taking a long deferred and much needed rest. But it seems that even in a womb fantasy there is danger attached, for if I satisfy myself with this form of feeding and body comfort, I shall be punished by being ejected.

In the dream I could not actually see what happened to the contents of the car, or who they were, but, if this is the punishment I am dreading, that would account for the fact that I could not see it clearly as myself being thrown out of the womb. Here I thought that whoever was tippled out of the car was not grossly damaged but only badly shaken, shocked, and probably bruised and *very* uncomfortable.

While in London I mentioned a desire to go shop-gazing. My whole attitude this time was, "Don't let us clutter ourselves up with business and other appointments, let us drift". The attraction in shop-gazing was to experience multi-colour sensations. That need again links up with what I have already said in relation to colour vibrations and all that which goes to the building-up of life while in the womb.

The windows displaying bright-coloured objects link up directly with No. 1 drawing of today where I am looking into the womb to experience once again, through the eye, these vibrations. The enact importance of the way in which one sense organ can deputise for the other senses is thus clearly demonstrated here. I have always been aware of a super-normal sensitivity of three of my sense organs, namely, touch, smell and sight. I believe I have, through my sight, kept a hold on life when otherwise it would have gone out. Throughout the analyses of R.M. and myself the colour hungers dominant in certain moods have been noted. These observations have led to the conviction that there is much relief to mental distress possible through colour-therapy.

Later that same day the following thought came, and I wrote it down because I felt it to be important.

"There is a mental assessment going on in the unconscious while in the womb. Everything is registered. The embryo or foetus is aware of every movement, Jerk, increase in pressure (intra-uterine) and sudden noise".

This thought is, as the next day's material will show, indicating the nature of the unconscious matter yet to be brought into consciousness. It indicates the eagerness of the unconscious to unload itself and to understand.

We now come to the following morning. Here are the notes written immediately on waking:

> I woke up with the words, "Golden Fleece", in my mind and thought, "What is the Golden fleece? I don't know. Anyway, it means this to me: something around one's body, so warm and light that one is not aware of it at all except as a pleasant sensation". My "Fuschia" painting then came to mind. This use a painting of a tiny flower-child in a sunny, enclosed space, looking down a long dark avenue of trees at the end of which is a spot of light. When this picture flashed into mind I thought, "It is warm where I am but looks exciting through the pin-hole at the far end of the tunnel".

There was something about Vesuvius in my dream. It is very vague. I think I was standing-by and giving warnings when what was going on became dangerous. "There are signs of Vesuvius in eruption" meant, "steady on there, you're arousing anger", or "Steady-you there, you are being too aggressive".

I was talking last night to R.M. and wondering why one should take birth as a punishment or, rather, what naughtiness the unborn or being-born infant could give itself as reason for the punishment of birth; for we know from this research that every hurt is argued by the infant into a punishment, and the reason why it is forced to come to this conclusion. A punishment can be avoided, an accident cannot. I thought, in answer to the above, that it is possible the foetus is aware of its aggression (even in utero) in its spasmodic kicks and that the throwing out of the womb at birth is taken as a punishment, not only because of being pushed out but because the manner of it is accompanied by compression and severe shock. The baby/me can only argue from the experience it has had, as follows:

> "Before I was always comfortable and happy. Now I am being attacked. Every few minutes I am being compressed to a state of blacking-out. I am gripped tightly on all sides. I cannot struggle or kick. It is a ghastly nightmare that has me in its grip and it goes on and on and never ends". (This feeling of things going on and on and on was a constant complaint throughout my analysis). In the passage through the bony pelvis the compression impedes the flow of blood and that is tantamount to the same feeling in a choking – "until things are blacked out".

The similarity between this and chokes makes me feel the birth re-experience will be the last I must go through. I still have a fear of being buried in a coffin. I always imagine myself in that ghastly position as suffocating to death and unable to move or to struggle. If one could struggle, even though one could not win, it would be easier than being held so that one could not struggle.

American psychologists experimenting on the reactions of infants to being held tightly have found that this action is resented more than any other.

After breakfast drawing was again resumed and continued after lunch. The notes on these drawings were written after a rest of a couple of hours, including tea. Here are the notes.

Within the main outline is myself. I am in the womb. The undulating line between myself and the womb wall, the main outline, indicates that the womb is attacking me at all points; compressing me. The drawing below this shows me being squeezed out into a long, thin tube. I am in the process of being born.

This is again attack from every point, and I am feeling gripped and held to suffocation point. My fear of being buried in a coffin comes into my mind at this moment.

At this point I felt the need of colour to get over what was wanted. Here I show myself being compressed and am bleached white as I am forced down into the canal. The blue indicates pressure.

The blue shapes in this picture are the attacking things. Attack is now definitely by compression as the base of each attacking instrument fits exactly to the outline of the womb (the red). My head and shoulders are in the canal, and I am compressed white and have blacked out. The thought that came to me while painting was, "I am blacking-out". I think the yellow in this picture is anticipating light in the outer world. The little purple half-moon shape in the left-hand bottom corner, at the top of the head, is the opening of the womb. The yellow cone below that is light.

I get the feeling that although I am blacking-out the blacking-out is coming and going in a concertina fashion. At this moment the thought, "This blacking-out came with every labour pain, that is with every fresh contraction of the uterus", flashed into my mind. I was puzzled by this yellow cone and purple half-moon shape because I felt while painting them that I was aware of this yellow as light impinging on my head and yet I was not sure for, at one moment I felt this was so and at the next that all was black; that is I was not aware of the light. It now becomes obvious that what happened was that with each compression I lost consciousness and was not aware of the light, and when consciousness came back, I was aware of it. I knew when I painted in the yellow cone that I was aware of light on the top of my head and, consciously, wished to put the yellow coming through the hole. But my unconscious would not allow it. It is now apparent why. It could not make the above point clear without the device of making the hole refuse the light as this picture is one in which the compression of the womb is in process. It is only during the interval of relaxation. between labour-pains that the sensation of light is experienced. I would like to mention here that there is data within the material of these "analyses" which I feel should throw light on the functioning of the Pineal body.

Here my head seems to have come through the tightest part of the canal and is about to come right outside. I am still colourless from compression but aware of a tremendous lot of light through the top of my head.

In this I appear to be well out. The strain of compression is removed, and some degree of colour is coming back. The background is all the blood and faeces and moisture that surrounds me. At this moment I think I am actually aware of these through smell and warmth.

Note that in this painting the umbilicus is shown for the first time in this set of paintings. No mention was made of this at the time of writing the notes, but it is referred to later.

When I had finished the last one, I thought it completed the series. Lunch came at this point. After lunch, when I sat down once more to draw, I was surprised and *bored* to find that I immediately did the outline of the baby figure again. I then did the circles, including that of the mouth, and thought, "All mouths screaming". The two detached feet seemed to have no meaning, nor all the ovals when they refused to be mouths; that is, when their colouring suggested they might be something else. I was not aware of the moaning of this picture until it was nearly finished. Naturally I was aware, because of the screaming mouth, that I was protesting against my arrival into the world. When I began putting in the black lines, I realised I was saying that I was being hurt at all points; and then the different types of hurts became conscious. The two blue discs are my hands which are "screaming" with pain as they come out of their numbness, which is indicated by the blue. The two green discs below indicate my legs, but I feel they have no feeling as yet. Nor have my feet which are a couple of dead lumps thrown anywhere. "Not being attached" means "not belonging", which, again means I am unaware of them. I am *faintly* aware of the legs (the green discs) but rather as numb lumps, which is possibly the reason for the use of green. My unconscious is saying, "My legs feel like lumps of number-two".

Throughout my analysis colours have had symbolic meanings, but that is another chapter of the research. Here, it must suffice to say that green has been used continually as a quality indicating excreta.

All the black marks on or near my body are smacks, stings. The red and black at the centre indicates that the pain *there* is sharper than elsewhere. This probably means that the severing of the umbilical cord is felt as a sharp pain. The four discs round the head I think indicate all the noises, touches and handling that is going on around me and impinging upon me. The two red arrows directed to my ear-holes are noises felt by me as sharp pain; stabbing and repeated as the arrow-heads are repeated. The purple stabbing angles on the top of my head I feel as "pins and needles"; such as I often get at night down the inner side of my arms (the blood pulsation), and which actually wakes me.

This feeling is what one gets after a part of oneself has been compressed and the blood has been kept out of a limb. It would seem from this as if one can experience "pins and needles" after the compression during birth.

After dictating the notes on these drawings, a state of exhaustion ensued, and I had a heavy sleep before supper and went to bed immediately after supper. This was an indication of extreme anxiety.

The next day's work again began with a dream. Its interpretation, which follows, was written immediately after breakfast.

I was dreaming, just before waking this morning. The dream was particularly detailed and vivid. A father, whose child had been drowned, felt convinced that a certain child called Marguerite had done it. There was a deep pit with a deep pool at the bottom. Several children had been missing lately. The father got hold of Marguerite and took her to the edge of this pit. He was determined to make her confess and then get rid of her by dropping her in. This is how he argued to himself:

> If I hand her over to the authorities, they will put her in a school for some years but will do nothing to understand what drives her to these deeds.

> They will not trouble to find out whether she is a hopeless lunatic or a curable subject. When she comes out again a number of useful citizens will be the price of the liberty of this lunatic. The authorities do not and will not protect. Therefore, I shall protect humanity from this curse and then drop out of life myself as I prefer this to being destroyed by the authorities.

The father took Marguerite to the pit and extracted from her, by the threat of swinging her over the pit by a rope and saying he would cut the rope if she didn't confess, the names of those she had destroyed and how she had done so. She gave the names of three she had destroyed (boys, I think, George was the name of one of them). She said she would be walking by the pit with the other child on the near side to the pit and then an uncontrollable impulse to give a sudden, strong, determined push would come. She had no reason for it. It was just a senseless push. The father then let go of the rope and got rid of Marguerite. He felt rather sorry but, the authorities being what they were, there was nothing else to be done. Partly in the dream still, but beginning to wake, I visualised the womb as I drew it yesterday and thought, "Yes! that's the pit; and being thrown into the pit is being thrown out of the womb. The senseless impulses of Marguerite are the senseless, sudden contractions of the womb which tipples the child over or out". I, the father in the dream, will protect all other children from being destroyed this way. I will destroy the attacking Marguerite. I am sorry because I realise somehow that Marguerite is a lunatic, that is a reasonless being subject to these impulses.

The child in the dream is walking along with Marguerite quite smoothly means the child is quite quiescent in the womb and then, suddenly, is attacked by a strong determined push.

I have always felt glad when a child has died. It has got away from the tragedy of life which I have felt as an agonising death-in-life. The whole of life has been a birth trauma repeated. In other words, I seem to have felt all the mental and emotional compression of my childhood as a repetition of the compression and consequent suffocation of childbirth.

I, the child being born, seem to have felt mentally the *reasonlessness* of the repeated attacks of the uterus. I lie there quiescent and then suddenly the attack comes and is repeated again and again. The compression impedes the blood flow through the umbilical cord and the feeling of suffocation takes place. The mind wants a reason for what happens for then a repetition can be avoided. If there is no reason one's position is desperate. The reason a child provides itself with is, "I am hurt (punished) because I attacked, therefore, I can stop these hurts by not attacking; but if there is no reason the case is desperate".

Yesterday I offered myself the suggestion that I probably thought the womb attacked me because I kicked inside. This, no doubt, I did. But my unconscious did not take this easy way out. It gave the whole agonising process of being born yesterday and then, in this dream, says the womb must be destroyed.

I am the father to the drowned children = father to myself. Note here the choice of method of destruction of the children, viz. by drowning. Drowning has been felt by me to be a suffocation.

My feeling of sorrow that Marguerite must be destroyed is due to the fact that Marguerite, the womb, is not all bad. I have a friendly feeling towards the womb as my warm, cosy cradle during pregnancy, but Marguerite the attacker must be destroyed so that no more children may be hurt that way. (I have identified all children with myself). In other words, the womb, as cradle, is not destroyed but the womb as attacker must be destroyed. Throughout life and analysis, I have frequently expressed my fear and hatred of reasonless attack.

It also explains the reason for my need that my basic theory, which is that the human is not basically a hating object but fundamentally and naturally capable of loving, should prove to be scientifically true. Hate, I maintain, is an effect and not an intrinsic quality of the human. I had to insist on that since if it were intentional attack, it was hate. Reasonless attack would then be intentional hate, which was unbearable. But intermittent contractions as a biological process is another matter. It is neither reasonless nor intentional hate.

I wondered why I put in the umbilical cord in drawing No. 6 of this series and had not done so before. I even thought at the time, "Shall I go over the others and put it in?" but my unconscious said "No". It seems that, as always, it was right. My umbilical cord was not put in before because its flow was being impeded and so, as far as I was concerned, was *not there*. After I had half emerged from the womb it must have started to pulsate again and, therefore, was once more there. My colleague and I, while writing up the notes on this painting, had noticed a change of colour in the face and body. The unconscious does not overlook a single detail.

The three boys mentioned in the dream probably refer to my mother's three previous births. Her womb had "killed" three times. How did the unconscious know this? I would not have the conscious knowledge of my mother's still-born first till I was probably about thirteen years old.

As we know, time does not exist in the unconscious. Subsequent knowledge would be assimilated by the unconscious and fitted into earlier events just as we consciously fit in early events and their consequences into later life. Here the later knowledge of my mother's still-born first is used when unconscious material relating to birth is coming up. After all it was only subsequent knowledge that allowed the unconscious to be aware of the other two births which had previously occurred. Another point is the accuracy of the unconscious. It never is inaccurate in statement of what it knows or has experienced.

I wondered why I called the womb Marguerite. "M" stands for mother, I thought, and then remembered that in my analysis I have frequently made children come out of flowers. Thus, a flower as a womb symbol was already present in the material of analysis but here it is singled out for specific purposes.

I remarked at this point that "the whole of a person's life is felt in terms of its very *first* trauma". I was realising that throughout life I had always felt limitations as a suffocation; as an impeding of the *flow* of life within me. And I was reflecting also as to whether my statement held good for others too.

In the case of my colleague, his first violent trauma was circumcision at eight days of age and throughout life he had reacted to all obstructions as attack on the *penis*. Further, the nature of the trauma colours the quality of the relief experienced at each realisation in consciousness of unconscious material. But I must not digress here as time does not permit.

The next day I did another series of drawings. Here are the notes.

This is me in the womb, opening out my legs and kicking vigorously. This is indicated by the zig-zag line proceeding from the feet.

Here I am kicking and stretching. The kicking takes place only where zig-zag lines occur, and where they do not appear I am stretching.

This is a repetition of the last, but the kicking is far more energetic. At this point I broke off to write, and here are those notes.

While I was doing this one, I got the thought, "Glory! I can stretch all my limbs at last with impunity", and then, "That's why I used to get an almost maniacal hate in the old days with the awful clogging of one's legs with the old-fashioned skirts. It represented the being held and compressed as a punishment". It also links up with my feeling that analysis goes on fer ever and ever and that nothing one does will ever make any difference. I must have thought, "It's because I kick that the womb is attacking me". But this was not so, for when I stopped kicking, even so, after an interval between labour-pains the womb would suddenly-attack without my kicking again; and this attack was repeated again and again. It does not matter how recent kicking may or may not have taken place. In the unconscious time does not exist. It knew it *had* kicked and that was the only thing it could catch hold of as a possible reason for the attack by the womb. This would constitute a reasonless attack as opposed to being attacked because of licking. It was infinitely preferable to be attacked for this reason because one could do something about it. One could stop kicking. But there was nothing to be done against reasonless attacks.

This accounts too for my inner distress when, in my childhood, I could not find myself guilty in the way demanded by the religion of my parents. If I could have felt guilty then I could have accepted their religion, but how was I to feel guilty for a reasonless repetition of attacks unrelated to kicking since I was no longer kicking. "Safe in the arms of Jesus" meant in my unconscious, "safe in the womb of mother". But when, for peace of mind, I contrived an emotional state of acceptance of this religion of Jesus and rested in his arms my conversion could not last for long as, almost at once, the unconscious fear of reasonless attack from those very arms, which symbolised the mother's womb, would arise. The thought, "I shall be doomed in the end and nothing I can do about it will make any difference", has always been at the back of my mind or inner consciousness. My life has been lived in the sense that one may as well be hanged for a sheep as for a lamb. In other words, whether I kick or not it makes no difference, and *kicking makes me feel the flow of life within me. It is stretching*. But although nothing stopped the womb from attacking me I must still have been uncertain and have thought my one time kicking started the attack. "To let myself full out", and "To experience life in every cell of my being", have been favourite phrases of mine. Thus, I have always kicked in life, that is, stretched; I have felt myself in all I have done, but always with the inner certainty I would be attacked and done to death by repeated suffocation in the end. That repeated suffocation, dying a thousand times, is explained by the repeated labour-pains which must have compressed the umbilical cord and brought about the blacking-out process.

During analysis, whenever I fantasied doing something which symbolically represented kicking or stretching or giving expression to myself, such as speaking on a platform to a group (which is making myself felt) I have anticipated attack. The feeling would be that the group would attack me, and I would be expulsed from it. Therefore, everything active or expressive of myself has been dangerous to me.

The birth trauma also explains why I have never been able to contemplate death as a finality. I have never been able mentally to assess death as having an end. The feeling and mental picture has been that one would go on and on suffocating to death without dying completely. Try as I would, I could not bring it to an end. In birth I was continually being brought back to life between labour-pains only to be battered and suffocated again to the point of losing consciousness. The words, "Leave me alone", so frequently written on earlier drawings, and the word, "Finis" on the drawing you have seen today were stating my wish not to come back to consciousness. They were the equivalent to saying, "Don't wake me up again and then batter and suffocate me to the blacking-out state again".

The phrase, "Running to death to escape death", which was often on my tongue has really meant, among other interpretations, a running to death to escape being born again. Death has simply meant the process of being born which, because of the position of my umbilical cord and the contractions of the uterus, was a repeated attack to the point of death with each labour pain. From this realisation I feel it becomes a matter of the utmost importance that accurate observations are made with regard to the details of the birth of every child. The child born after a few labour-pains will not experience a trauma of this kind but the child of a long labour, or with a twisted umbilical cord, or from a mother with a small or contracted pelvis may well result in a psychological trauma which will cause much suffering throughout life.

While recently thinking over the question of speaking in public (which, you will remember, is comparable to actively expressing the flow of life within me), I have felt that I could read a paper with comparative freedom from anxiety so long as there was no question time. Question time would destroy me. I would not be able to understand the questions. There is, of course, a reality situation. Having been so long away from the analytic atmosphere, both in reading and attending meetings, I should not be able to understand the highly technical and rapidly increasing language with its hair-splitting variations. But that did not account for the intensity of the fear of these questions. The fear was that under the stream of questions my mind would "blank out". It seems to me that I must have felt that my kick was the first attack and had initiated the contraction of the womb. So, I am saying: "If I could give a lecture without questions, that is to say without initiating an attack, I am free now of all my other fears in relation to speaking in public; but if I allow questions I shall blank out". This is taking the question itself as an attack which suffocates to the point of blacking-out. (The work of the super-ego in relation to this is obvious but cannot be amplified now).

Being able to answer a question is being able to pacify the attacker. In the womb I found there was no way of pacifying the attacker. To stop the kicking and lie still did not pacify. The fear in being unable to answer a question seems to lie in the feeling that I shall not be able to pacify and then I shall be attacked and expelled from the group, i.e. from the mother's womb.

When I began drawing and found myself depicted as definitely kicking in the womb my conscious self said, "Well! You know all about that. Why do you now have to draw it?" and its immediate response was, "You are now allowing yourself satisfaction in what has long been withheld from you because you now know you will not be attacked (punished) and that kicking was not naughty".

Thus, I immediately and symbolically experience the relief I have so long needed.

Throughout life I have always slept with my knees drawn almost up to my chin. Recently, after a previous piece of analysis, I was able to stretch out in bed. But during this present bout of analysis, I have been sleeping huddled up again. This seems to me to be due to the coming up of this last bit of analytic revelation. While huddled up I could avoid kicking which was dangerous to me until I realised that the womb was not punishing me for kicking. I may add here that since this I seldom find myself sleeping huddled up as before.

After supper on this day, I went to bed and played Patience. I expressed my feeling and condition as being tired but not exhausted: a different sort of tiredness. I wanted a lazy form of amusement and without any sort of exertion.

The next morning, I was up early and very active. First did a little gardening. After this I had the feeling of wanting to paint in oils but at the same time was not pleased at this as I thought I had finished my analysis the day before.

Actually, yesterday's work was the completion of the birth trauma but my unconscious, now that it was finding release from its most disturbing fears, was anxious for further alleviation. The material that follows is related to what followed immediately after the birth which, in the unconscious, is essentially part and parcel of the birth-trauma.

It distressed me to think that there seemed still more to come. But it had to be done so I began to draw with pencil. My unconscious, however, demanded oils so I gave in and painted with oils. I did two oil paintings, one after the other. Here are the notes on the first pencil drawing and the two oils.

This is me stretching. In my body, in the lower right portion of it, is drawn an eye and underneath it is the letter "I", followed by the word "wake". Thus, the drawing is saying I wake and stretch.

I drew in the outline and thought, "It's me stretching again". To my surprise I painted the whole thing in as flowers and leaves. All the background is water. I am stretching inside the womb. The red flower is the seat of warmth and is placed where the umbilicus comes into my body, which is green and striped with orange. My legs are green and marked with red stripes, and they are kicking. My pink leaf-arms are twisting, turning and stretching.

This painting was done quickly; in just over an hour.

Immediately upon finishing the last painting I began on this one. The horned cow-head in bottom left corner is a mother animal. The yellow disc in the midst of the grassy foliage represents me. The tongue going from the cow's head to two dark discs on me is the umbilical cord feeding me through the umbilicus (lower disc) and my mouth (top disc). The two larger red discs on either side are my ears and the numerous black arrows going into the centre of each indicate a battering noise. The red crosses above are saying that all this noise hurts my head. While painting this the thought was in my mind that the cow was bellowing and that I was saying, "If it would only stop bellowing and hurting me with the noise it could then feed "me with its long tongue". I realised later that the long tongue to feed my mouth was what I expected since it was a long-tongued-umbilical cord which fed my belly-mouth (umbilicus) when I was in the womb. The green grass, I think, is the cow's food. I think the bellowing of the cow may have been my mother's groans during labour. My last picture of yesterday's series indicated the pain of noise at the time of birth – *outside* the womb. This painting represents the idea of being inside the womb and as the thought, "If only the cow would stop bellowing and feed me", was in my mind, it seems obvious I am trying to get back to the time before the bellowing began.

The reason I had to paint in oils today is that I can be *more vigorous* with that medium; and this, I think, symbolises a fighting with my limbs against everything that is impinging upon me in this re-experience of the birth trauma.

I feel, at this point, it is important to remind you again that no notes were written at the time and, while painting, I was only very partially aware of what was coming up.

After an interval for tea, I started painting again but this time in watercolour. Here are their notes.

Having stated, in the previous painting, that I wish to be back in the womb I seem now to be proceeding to say why. This is me with my mouth open and yelling. The reasons are manifold: I am being bathed, as shown by the blue; all the noises hurt my head, denoted by the red arrow-heads; but the thing that hurts more than anything else is the iron band of the nurse's hands round my legs (the ring of red) as she pulls me up to wash my bottom, or smack it, for red arrows indicate pain there too. The patchiness and colour of my legs conveys the fact that they are partially numb and in a state of "pins and needles".

This is myself, still being bathed. The red band, which indicates the hand holding my legs, is the principle point of pain. The cut umbilical cord and my bottom are also hurt. I seem to realise that my mouth is making a noise which hurts my ears. This is conveyed by the arrows coming from the red issuing from my mouth.

I am still being bathed but feel I am getting quieter. The sharpness of the umbilical pain is dying down and the pain from the noise of my crying is lessening with my diminishing cries. One pain still remains. The fierce grip on my legs.

Here I am being dried and still crying; but much less. There is no longer that cruel grip of the red ring round my ankles. I am now objecting to the roughness of the towel or the hands that rub me with the towel.

I was very tired of these baby paintings and wondered if I would be quicker with pencil. The top left outline is myself throwing my limbs about in protest and my mouth is yelling its protest as shown by the radiating lines from the circle which is the mouth. The curly shape below this, which ends with a fringe of lines to the right, is the towel against which I am protesting. The circle to the right is the womb with me inside it. Thus, I am saying, "I hate this being dried which hurts me. Let me get back to peace in the womb".

I thought that after being dried it was the finish but here my unconscious is again protesting against being hustled and smothered. The pink shape is me on the blue towel on the nurse's lap. The mass of green is the general feel of the nurse's body. The blue and red of the background and the shape like a pair of sugar-tongs are the nurse's moving arms which seem to keep up a general battering of me. I feel smothered with these arms and hands. My life is being nearly battered out of me by the way the nurse keeps on pulling my legs over my head to attend to my bottom.

In the last two days I have gone to bed immediately after supper, feeling too tired and exhausted to do anything else. Last night I was not so exhausted as the night before that but wanted to be allowed to lie still and make no effort. I noticed that all yesterday I felt very passive and quiescent. This was plainly resistance to what was about to emerge, i.e. the molestation by the nurse. Today, and while doing these notes, I feel very irritable and want to scream at the slightest interference which, of course, again fits in with what has been coming through today. Every remark of R.M.'s seemed to batter me. It also connects up with my irritation, throughout analysis, at his attempts to push things or make me go his way. It has made me very irritable. Furthermore, my sensitiveness to sound, and the pain in my head and ears as a result of this, explains my anger with him when he raises his voice in a loud fashion whenever he becomes excited or insistent. I invariably use the phrase, "Stop buggering me", when he is on his forcing tactics and, in this set of paintings, it is my bottom which is mainly being attacked.

Again, the next day's work began with a dream. Here are the notes:

Dreamt of R.M. and myself, in the little Austin, and a woman friend and her mother in another car, motoring. We went down a narrow street and lost sight of the other car. Something went wrong with our car. We all then found ourselves in a lady's house: a very grand dame and house. R.M. seemed disinclined to see to the car and quite excited by this dame's entertainment, not realising how bored she was at having to entertain such riff-raff, as we seemed to her. The servants and other members of the household did not trouble to keep their feelings of disgust and contempt from their faces and, in some cases, from their remarks. R.M. was too dull-witted to realise what was going on. The rest of us were consumed with discomfort and a longing to get away. But we were dependent on my companion to get us away and he was absorbed with the old lady. I stared out of countenance a man who made an insulting remark. We finally got away and R.M. went on in advance to the garage to fetch the car. We walked in the direction he had gone, but somehow he contrived to miss us. I thought, "Oh my god! He's gone back to that cursed house". I found him there and he said the car had gone wrong again. He brought it into the drawing-room and asked me to stand on a sofa and hold it up on end so that he could get at a part for greasing. Then he went away again. I was in a frantic state, for I could not move with this thing in my hands, and I was terrified the unpleasant people of the house would come and make rude remarks. The servants were coming and going and sniffing contempt. At last, he came again. He had forgotten he had left me there and had gone wandering round the house out of curiosity. I thought him the dullest-witted imbecile and the thickest-skinned person I had ever met. I was savage with him. I got him and the car out of the house at last. But I was still on tenterhooks as we had to tinker with the car just outside the house. The people coming from and going to the house were bound to notice us and when they saw we were the interlopers of yesterday they would certainly attack us. Yesterday they could not in the presence of their hostess, who, by treating us with civility, demanded an outward show of it from the others. R.M. argued with me, saying the hostess was quite pleased to have us there. I explained that she was only being courteous because it was her house and her social code to act so and that as soon as we were gone there would be an outburst of the vilest epithets hurled at us: and the hostess would express her feelings in two or three words; she would speak of us as "those peculiar people" in a tone of voice as if for the first time she had met with a garden slug and pushed it with her toe out of curiosity. That was the dream.

Thinking about it after breakfast I suddenly realised its interpretation.

Contempt is always associated with contempt of something smelly and dirty. My analysis is concerned at the moment with the various unpleasant and painful things which were experienced by me at birth. I think the dream is a protest against the awful faecal stench that surrounded me before being washed for the first time. This stench must have been a violent new stimulation after birth. My olfactory organ would be stimulated for the first time with the onset of respiration, and any violent stimulation constitutes attack.

Having to get out of the car and leave it to be repaired is being turned out of the womb.

I dreaded painting in oils yesterday and remarked to this effect saying, I was afraid I would have to do some though I hated the thought of it. Oil paint has always meant faeces in my unconscious.

Going back to yesterday's oil paintings: I disliked the green body and legs I gave myself in the first oil painting and also the whole picture. It gave me the feeling of being rather muddy coloured. (Green, we must remember, stands for faeces.) I actually said at the time that I did not like any of the colouring of these two oils. So in the first of these paintings, I am being bathed after birth but dislike the unpleasant stimulation my olfactory nerve is receiving. The background is the bathwater which is rather dirty.

In the second oil painting I felt that my interpretation had left out something important and I was also slightly dissatisfied with the interpretation of the tongue as the umbilical cord. I felt it had some additional meaning – that the interpretation was not finished. I experienced this same feeling with regard to interpreting the green grass as food. Furthermore, I wanted to put a lot of brown into the grass but could not do it because I thought I should spoil it if I did. I also felt there was something to say about the background but could not get at anything at the time.

Referring now to the umbilical cord again: the upper prolongation I now feel is going to the nose (previously mentioned as a mouth) and the lower to the mouth (previously mentioned as the umbilicus). I think it is stating the wish that I was fed by the umbilical cord into my nose and mouth because the food that I got from the umbilical cord was not repellent and frightening like the food, that is the unpleasant smells and tastes, that was coming through my nose and mouth at that time of my being born (and later while being bathed). The green grass, interpreted yesterday as cow-food, is really excreta which seemed to smother me when I was born. Calling it cow-food was the nearest interpretation I could bear in consciousness but it nevertheless symbolised the real thing since baby-excreta has been mother-food previously in analysis. To describe it as mother-food and paint it green (my colour for baby-excreta) was all I could manage yesterday, though another part of me knew I wanted it mainly brown and yellow, i.e. grown-up excreta. The little brown and yellow colour I succeeded in putting in was by a great effort and did not please me.

And now to return to the dream.

Apparently, the car is finished and ready for me again, but somehow I miss it. This seems almost as if the mother's bed was ready for me and the general mess cleaned up, for being outside the house means I am outside the zone of contempt and disgust; that is of smell. But somehow the car is missed, and I find myself back in the house once more and R.M. once again saying the car is out of order.

This time the car is inside the house and R.M. tells me its back-end must be greased. I stand on a sofa and hold it nearly upside down so that he can get at it. I am left in that position. The interpretation of this is that before reaching the mother's bed again, that is the renovated car, I find myself back in the same position of stink and contempt as before. This time the car stands for a nappy and, I think, holding the car up-ended on the couch means myself being held up-ended while my bottom is being seen to; cleaned up and greased. R.M., in the dream, had wandered off and left me in this appalling position. "Yes!" I thought, "while nurse (that is R.M.) is hunting around for the necessaries with which to deal with me". An uncomfortable position like that will feel endless to a new-born babe.

In this part of the dream, I am terrified that the contempt (=stink) will accumulate and distress me as before, but at this point there is only a little stink for there were only one or two contemptuous servants about. Most of the people there in the first place who were around me and smothering me, (the doctor, nurse and other attendants at my birth) were absent. This would also be saying that all the faecal matter, blood and general mess that was assailing my nostrils and mouth in the first instance were absent. But, in the dream, I was in a state of frenzy lest an attack of faecal odour should reach me again before I got outside and away in the clean car (=back in the mother bed), which also symbolised the mother-womb, or any place of clean, non-smelling comfort.

I think what actually must have happened at birth was that I was bathed and freed from the attack of smell and set aside in a clean warm blanket. But I did not reach the car (the mother-bed). After a time, I am found by the nurse again because, once more, there is a stink. I have made a stool in my nappy: I am back in the house of stink.

After an endless time R.M. (the nurse) returns and tells me the car has broken down again. The car this time is myself, but I have not yet differentiated between the mother and myself. The nurse cleans me up and finally I am outside again, outside the house of stink.

The mother of my woman friend seems to represent the grand dame of the house, that is the clean person. I think that bringing them into the dream is recalling the fact that my mother and I were clean and free from this dirt and stink attack previously, before birth, because although my friend and her mother, that is my mother and myself, come into the house there was nothing in the dream to indicate that their car had broken down. They were merely waiting for our car to be set right. This suggests that my mind was not fully adjusted to what had happened. When I was cleaned up, quiet, and rolled in a blanket, or in the mother-bed, I was still in the mother-womb (so I thought) and, that being so, it was not my car (=my friend's and mother's car) that had broken down. The realisation is that when I am clean I am in the intact car, as clean daughter of the clean mother, but when I am dirty I an outside the clean car (=the mother-womb) and in a dirty nappy (=the car that breaks down); that is, every time I smelt myself or my dirty nappy I became awake to the fact that I was no longer inside the mother.

This same morning, soon after the writing of the interpretation of this dream, I started on painting again (the large water-colour painting). I was aware of its meaning to a large extent when I had completed it, but I did not get down to its interpretation until the material, which follows, had been brought up. This had to be dealt with first as thoughts in relation to it completely possessed my mind to the exclusion of all else at this moment. Here are those notes:

It occurred to me that the birth shock to my olfactory nerve should have some connection with the sudden resurrection of my fear of lecturing which came up again yesterday. In the picture I have just painted I have confined the nurse with all the stink and blood, with which I have been attacked, to the corner of the picture. If I am bullied and battered with questions and contempt (=stink) it is more than I can stand. It is frightening and terrifying. Not understanding complicated language (a constant fear) here means not understanding the faecal attack. I shall be completely smothered and helpless against that sort of language and, when I think of being questioned, I always think of people who discharge words of this complicated type at the rate of a machine gun. Simple language is clean language. Complicated language is a bad smell. If I am smeared with that language I shall be overwhelmed by the insufferable stench. Contempt, and a thing for which one holds contempt, seem both to have the same meaning. Contempt is the thing thrown at you for being dirty later, just as it was at the time of birth. Since the primitive only knows one law, namely, "an eye for an eye and a tooth for a tooth", contempt and faeces become one and the same thing.

If I want to secure a comfortable place within a womb (=be accepted in any group) I have to go through a birth situation; that is go back through the process by which I came. One of the birth shocks was the attack by smell (= questions = fear of contempt).

I do not know if my olfactory organ is unduly developed or whether many children suffer a psychological trauma in this respect. At any rate this material serves to show how necessary it is to consider every detail in relation to the birth of a child and to make the birth and subsequent cleaning of the child as quickly, gently and considerately as possible.

All through the painting of these oils, and while I painted the large watercolour, I experienced foul smells in my nostrils. So great was my anxiety that I could not even consider, at that time, the possibility of them being of psychological origin. Subsequently this was realised when the smell entirely disappeared after these realisations came up. Furthermore, I have always been ultra-sensitive to smells and it was a matter of amazement to my professors, in the viva examination in Materia Medica as a student, when they could not find a single drug which I could not instantly name after the merest sniff.

Here is something further in relation to lecturing. If I cannot answer questions, it means I am not grown-up (=have no knowledge) and that means I am a baby. It is babies that are attacked with faeces (=contempt).

To call a person a baby is synonymous with calling them smeared with faeces since it is usually used as a contemptuous phrase. One does not wish to have these forcible reminders of the repellent shock of faecal contamination at birth.

And now for the notes on the large watercolour.

Needless to say, the figure of the baby is myself, in water, swimming away to dive under the blue and orange horse-shoe-shaped thing in the left lower corner. I have only given myself a mouth and have supplied myself with the food and warmth that I was previously accustomed to receive through the umbilicus. The umbilical cord is in my mouth and trailing from it is the womb which I carry away with me in fantasy. I am pulling it out of the mother (the large pink shape at top right) and its feet and arms indicate it needs a lot of pulling; that it doesn't want to come. Its feet are checking the movement towards me caused by my pulling. In the right-hand bottom corner is a black bird with its claws and feelers surrounding an enormous mass of blood and faeces. The bird is nurse. She is welcome to all the blood and faeces as I wish to get away from that filthy odour which my last pictures show as causing me acute distress.

The blue circle with the yellow centre, to the left of my head, is my mouth eager for milk (yellow). But as milk is not forthcoming, I revert to the umbilical cord. The weakness of the milk colour gives me the feeling that I hardly was able to sense milk as such and as coming from the mother. In any case it was insufficient. The curling blue lines just above and to the right of this indicates the currents of the water. I think by the water I am saying, "I like the warmth of the water in the womb". The blue horse-shoe shaped thing under which I am diving I think are the bedclothes. The orange is flickering daylight. Thus, the whole picture is saying,

> If my mother won't have me, I don't mind being in this new bed, or new womb, if I can carry my old womb along with me and, particularly, my supply of food and warmth. What I have no use for at any price is the nurse with her blood and faeces.

The water is fresh and clean from any taint of faeces or blood.

When my colleague asked the reason for the size of this painting I said, "It gives me room to move around in. I am not cramped by clothes".

No drawing was done the next day as I felt I needed rest. The notes with regard to that day were as follows:

I had an overwhelming sleep between lunch and tea today. I realised that I could give way to it without keeping one ear open all the time, so to speak, as I have usually done, but was soaking in it as I have never been able to before. This is a new type of sleep: heavy and soggy. I am also astonished at my freedom to indulge in sleep as usually I should feel it was a desperate waste of time.

When my associate, R.M., dropped something in the kitchen just now I did not feel the need to attack him for being careless, that is dirty.

I realise now that my insistence that people should be clean, tidy and capable is a protective measure against being attacked with dirt; in other words, I won't have people around me who attack with dirt.

I noticed just now that instead of undergoing that hopeless feeling in relation to getting R.M. to be anything but a dirt attacker, that is the dirty nurse, I thought, "Poor fellow. I expect he is tired".

Just before supper, while in my bath, I had the fantasy of being endowed liberally with money for our work (for a clinic) and, separately, for ourselves too, liberally. The two outstanding points in this fantasy were that by the liberal, personal endowment, in addition to funds for a clinic, one could satisfy every-whim in the short vacations one would take. This meant that every hunger-ridden sense could be satisfied. The other thing for which the money would be expended would be for getting knowledge, whenever it became necessary, in the quickest possible and most easily understood way. Not understanding is an intolerable situation. As long as a thing is not understood it is reasonless and reasonless attack is dangerous. Therefore, understanding must be given as quickly as possible the moment the need arises. I thought at this point, "If my mother had been able to feed me satisfactorily after my birth it would have alleviated the idea that attack is the only and the inevitable end of all things". In the fantasy, a lack in the chain of knowledge must be immediately supplied and knowledge, in one of its aspects, is food. The fact that my mother had little, or no milk, must have meant at least a few days of hunger since it was accompanied by indigestion and vomiting. Earlier analysis had brought this fact to light, and also that the vomiting had been taken as attack.

The satisfaction of all one's hunger needs in respect of comfort, colour, smell, warmth and food, is what one requires immediately after the strain of work. Work, here, meaning being born.

These notes, as you will have gathered, show that awareness of freedom from unconscious strain and anxiety, and of the assimilation of what has been brought into consciousness, is speedily taking place.

Although rest from drawing and analysis was still my intention, the dream that came through the next morning was attended to and its interpretation speedily brought to light. Here it is.

In the dream last night, I met E.J. He showed me some photographs. He said he was retiring unless he I could entirely go his own way. Waiting on another person I for committee meetings was too much a strain when that person seldom turned up. I sympathised with him. While looking at the photos I said, "I can see them but not very clearly without my glasses; but my sight is vastly improved. I worked on the Bates method you know". I said this as he looked at me. His look seemed to say, "you are only pretending to look at those photos, you can't really see them as you haven't your glasses". In the dream I was surprised to find that I was actually seeing the photos far clearer than I actually can in waking life, as my eyesight, even with the glasses I am wearing, has been much worse lately". That was the dream.

E.J., in the dream, seems an identification with myself. "Waiting on another person ... was too much strain", seems waiting for a nurse and, therefore, food; and the waiting for food was, apparently, too much of a strain because I am sympathising with E.J. His doubt that I see without glasses, that is without outside help, is saying, "You cannot do what you want to do, go away (wide large water-colour) without outside (=nurse's) help".

It struck me, on thinking this over, that perhaps my unconscious was seeing things clearer than I yet do in consciousness: that this might be the interpretation of my dream; that I was, in fact, seeing more clearly in the unconscious than I yet knew.

I was pleased with this dream as it clearly showed that my unconscious had assimilated and accepted the realisations I have made so far, but that there was still something more to be brought to light before my vision would be absolutely clear – that is before my analysis would be complete.

During the last few days, I have been dull and heavy with sleep and without sensation of strain. This feeling is comparable to the way one collapses into an inert lump when a long-continued strain is ended. It is interesting that this morning I woke early. Recently I have slept heavily till awakened. I feel inert but no longer dull and heavy.

I also noticed this morning that, for the first time for a long time, I enjoyed my breakfast. My taste felt fresh and clean to my food, was how I thought of it. I had not been enjoying my food lately for my taste seemed as if it had been dirtied and, therefore, I could not get the pleasure of the clean food given me. This so fits in with the re-experiencing of the befoulment of birth, in the last bit of analysis, that it must be the interpretation. My realisation of freedom will only come gradually into consciousness in these ways.

Nothing more was done this day. This point in the analysis marks the completion of the afterbirth trauma.

The whole of the day following was passed without any form of analysis – a complete rest: a pause for assimilation. The following was noted down.

I have been very inert; mentally asleep. I have actually slept off and on during a considerable part of the day. Tonight, I had a bath and did not lie and soak and daydream, or work out problems as usual, but came out almost at once.

The feeling of hurry, of wanting things to happen quickly in my analysis, seems to have gone, or is in abeyance.

And now for the next day's notes when work was resumed. Here they are.

In my dream last night, I went to a strange town and found a room in an hotel. I left my things there and went out. Then I found myself in an hotel with my family. Later, on leaving the town, I went to get my things from the first hotel but could not find the place again. I eventually found myself in a women's club, asked for the lavatory and was shown a place with only curtains drawn across the opening. I felt annoyed at the publicity but sat down. A nurse came along and said, "I'll help you", and poked me hard in the stomach. I said, "that hurts. Don't do that! I can manage". A little boy was running around playing and a man was cutting bread and butter, or something of that kind, at the table. When he put the knife down, he stuck it in the wood of the table, not seeming to realise that he had cut the table-cloth in doing so.

I could not make much of the dream. The hotel, where the family was, is probably the drawing-room. My clothes had been left elsewhere, possibly taken off as I come in from a walk. The lavatory scene seems plainly laid in the nursery.

I am still feeling very sleepy and dull mentally and seem to drift on.

That completes the dream notes.

Until noon I gardened and then came in not knowing what I was going to do. I still felt drifting. On sitting down at my desk, I began to play with paint and found myself painting. I continued to do so till 8.30 p.m., when I settled down to notes. Feel slightly more awake now but still very "laissez faire".

Here are the notes on the drawings just mentioned:

This is me. I feel I am being carried. I have a bunch of brightly coloured things in my hands. The blue and mauve around me is my cot. My posture makes me feel I am being lifted out of it. The two blue eyes and the faint outline of blocks, to the right, seem all that my eyes are seeing. My face is older than my usual baby faces and has a rather far-away-not-there look. I think the flowers are merely the sensation of many colours around me.

This is me as flower-buds, all unopened. That means I am not yet awake. The blue and dark green below is the soft, solid warmth of a lap beneath me. This is so because the two leaves above my head in the yellow sky are eyes and where those of a nurse would be if I were on her lap.

This gives me a feeling of being in bed with mother. I am the yellow bird and mother the red animal underneath me. The blue donkey may be my elder brother in father's arms. Father is the green animal.

The yellow line is the edge of my cot against the light. The brown circles are eyes looking in at me. The blue line is myself and its point signifies my eyes looking at the eyes which are looking at me. The three-pronged claw on the blue line is to show my hand is useless and cannot take hold of those eyes. Only my eye can hold them.

This again is the effect of eyes which I get looking in at me while I am lying in my cot.

This again I feel I am seeing from the cot. They are black, fearsome fingers. The circle I feel is a mirror on the wall reflecting a window. The tall brown window to the right of this is both a window and a door. Where the lower part of this meets the ground, it is purple and light, and this is because it meets the cot edge. The green Spot on the hand, to the left, may be a spectral spot – green being complementary to red. The wavy lines indicate the movements of colour of which I was aware.

Here again I feel I am representing what I am seeing from a lying position. An arm with three eyes attached, the corner of drawers with a series of four cushions of sorts lying on it and, to the left, what I think represents folded eyeglasses on a black cord.

Here are eyes and mouths peering down at me. The oval containing line is the opening of my cot. The two fingers to the left are holding on to the cot to look in and I think are my brother's who is being allowed to take his first look at me.

The oval contour is again the opening to my cot. The blue, black and purple indicate it is night and all is darkness out of the immediate neighbourhood of light. The yellow, green and blue object with the red centre, to the left, is probably a chandelier. The red and orange waves of colour is the firelight flickering on the ceiling and walls.

In all these paintings I seem to be recording my first experiences of being awake. I feel entirely passive, half awake and enjoying colour movement. Eyes are attracting me because of the scintillation. In fact, most of today's paintings have scintillating colour.

It is apparent that the unconscious, at this stage of the recording of its experiences and their sequence, has reached a moment when pain and molestation from the nurse are no longer present and it is unhampered in its pleasures in new experiences.

I had enjoyed doing this last series. I felt that now I could really take a rest from analysis. The decision to stop analysis, to take a good rest and to get back to the work of compiling the book was made.

On reflecting on today's work it appears to me that the appreciation of kaleidoscopic effects started as soon as my eyes were opened. This is clear from the drawings which you have just seen which describe my awareness of the new surroundings after I wake from the first sleep.

The acuity of sensations, the registration of every sensation as a stored memory and the fact that each experience of any sensation is built up and into all that constitutes the mental essence of any individual is not only here clearly defined and demonstrated, but its detail is comparable to the microscopic definition of each separate cell that goes to form the whole body of the individual.

Analysis, three months previously, had connected the kaleidoscope with chandelier-prisms. Now the time of this primary experience is given, namely, after my very first sleep.

But the unconscious had more to relate. There was yet another fear, related to the birth trauma, which was revealed the next day. On this day leisure and pleasure filled the hours until 9 p.m. when, as my notes will now relate:

In a pause during card-playing, while listening to the wireless news, I started scribbling on a pad.

The first was a quick scribble portrait of R.M., using him as the model. The second was R.M. again, but not using him to draw from, and was a deliberate attempt at making the face as ugly as possible. In other words, destroying it. The eye-lashes and curved lines in the forelook, and the lines from the ears, were put in later and, interpreted, means "the person concerned with 'pissing'". I then put in the line enclosing our card scores and then thought, "This is my cot". The legs below, attached to the bottom enclosing line, means "the cot that walks". So perhaps it is my pram. The raised leg in the bottom right corner of this shape is kicking mud (= "er-er") off me. The head peering over the cot, with one of the two eyes extended, is staring into my two eyes which are the two noughts of the card scores. This is shown by the arrows directed to the two noughts. At this moment I became aware that I was poisonously hating doing it. However, I kept on. The object directly below this, marked (4), is myself, "pissing" and "shitting" into the top oval shape which is a cot. At the last moment I gave the cot a leaf-shaped body and legs (below) with which to run away. At this stage I became aware of myself shivering and of an internal whimper of fright. It took me all my time to carry on. I realised that some unconscious fear was rising and had to force myself to "let go" to it. The dark lizard-like creature at the top right corner, marked (5), came next but began only as a scribble. It was a "pizz" and "shit". Its conversion into an animal shape was to blot out the rising discomfort.

In the next drawing, the scribble marked (1) is a "pizzing" and "shitting" again. I became aware that all the rest of the scribbles on this sheet were indicating the same thing and that all the subsequent decoration of the scribbles was camouflage; an indication of extreme anxiety; I was making a mess and I was terrified.

This is the same again: myself, "pizzing" and "shitting". At the bottom I accept the situation without camouflage and just scribble a mess. As I felt like stopping, R.M. pressed me to carry on and I responded by saying, "It hurts".

Here I do the same again. This is the mess I am making.

All the while I was drawing the shivering and whimpering was increasing, and suddenly I felt I wanted to scream and scream in terror. I asked for a bath to be got ready quickly and while I was left alone in the room, I let myself go still further: shivering and crying and making little screams. I was shuddering all over. When in the bath, my face and hands began twitching. I gave myself up to this until I understood its significance.

Previous to this happening I had, for some days, been in a state in which I was hardly awake and had periodically dropped on a couch, or my bed, and slept heavily. I had, at first, attributed this heavy sleeping to relaxation; the exhaustion following the lack of relaxed sleep. (Very light sleep has been usual with me throughout adult life). Yet I felt there was something wrong with the nature of this sleep for it did not refresh me, as it should have done, and seemed to be developing into a physically exhausting type of sleep. I was terribly reluctant to admit to myself that there was something else to come up for analysis for, having brought into consciousness the birth trauma, I felt it should be the end; and so was resisting the idea that the slumber was anything but a relaxation.

When I came in from the garden to prepare supper today I was feeling utterly unable to keep awake. I took a restorative and lay down for a while in order to wake myself up. At this stage I accepted the fact that my condition was a psychological exhaustion, and that further analysis was necessary.

While in the bath, which I took immediately after the drawings, I realised that my face and hand twitching was the re-experiencing of my muscular reactions to the re-awakening of the birth trauma.

Eyery time I "wee-weed" or "er-ered" in my cot, which was my symbolic womb, I was ruthlessly taken out again; torn out of it and attacked. I was hauled out, thumped and banged about and my legs were held in that biting grip. This all happens in the process of cleaning me up and putting on a clean nappy. With every movement, whether in changing the dressing or in the movement of the dressing when jarred by the hands on my body, my umbilical cord gave me piercing, sharp pains. This links up with yesterday's dream where the nurse prodded and gave me sharp pains in the stomach while I was making a stool, and father hurting me (poking me in the umbilicus) while I was being fed (the knife stabbing the table-cloth). It explains also the meaning of adding the leaf-body and the legs to the incident depicted in drawing No. 1 where, after urinating and defecating into the cot, I give it legs with which to run off; obviously so that nurse should not discover I had dirtied my nappy and, therefore, commence attacking me.

Further the destruction of R.M. in the second drawing, where I make him as ugly as I can, is the destruction of nurse; a necessary procedure to relieve me from my fears.

Thus, every waking after my birth became a re-enactment of the birth trauma and was associated with acute pain, a general banging about and a shivering from cold.

While painting the day before I noticed the reappearance of the nasty smell, which I had experienced some days back, while painting. My morning coffee had been drunk on that day without the slightest recollection later in the morning of having had it. It had a nasty taste, that is an "er-er" taste, and I had suppressed the memory of it. Today again my taste has been bad, and I left my evening coffee after the first sip. I had also been conscious of great reluctance in relation to doing anything. This "doing" meant making a stool or "wee-weeing". All these incidents indicate the gradual and forcible emergence into consciousness of the re-experience of the unpleasantness which was associated with each attack by the nurse in cleaning me up.

Summing up: my unconscious, the baby me, registered the fact that wet and smell were always accompanied by attack from the nurse, and this was associated with acute pain. The skin of the new-born infant with its natural sensitiveness and pressure sensitivity, which had not previously felt anything more rough or sharp than water (amniotic fluid), has not, perhaps, been given sufficient consideration hitherto. The roughness of the nappy, the soreness of the umbilical cord and rough handling can produce pain to the extent of shock in a new-born baby; and anything that can minimise these original traumata will help considerably in determining the child's future psychological attitude towards life.

Another point that came up was the meaning of card-playing, which, at my express wish, has frequently been played recently. Card-playing demands no mental effort. No more than pushing marbles about and enjoying the changing colour pattern. Card-playing is not working, that is not making a stool, and, therefore, safe from attack.

Again, the remarkable dream of three days back, where I see photographs more clearly than in day-life, comes to mind. This dream was the medium by which my unconscious was conveying to the conscious me that though it, the unconscious, understood the birth trauma better (more clearly) than did the conscious self in waking life, it was aware also of the clearing process that had yet to follow. It clearly demonstrates the unrelenting persistence of the unconscious in demanding that *every* item be explained and understood, and its thoroughness in attaining its purpose.

As a result of some earlier analysis, I had been thinking, previous to this birth trauma coming up, of lecturing freely as of something that could now be done without distress or faltering. But since the emergence of the birth material, I have felt rising in me once again the thought that I might not be able to lecture. I was becoming less and less sure of my ability to do so. Previous analysis has shown lecturing to be a "wee-weeing" and "er-ering" in public, amongst other things. My aim and hope has always been that I can produce something so clearly put, so complete, that I should be absolutely safe from attack. In other words, that I can produce something so clean that there would not be a dozen nurses – questioners – rising up in the lecture hall to tear me to bits. To be inadequate to the occasion, to have insufficient knowledge, is to be in a position of not being able to look after oneself, that is unable to be clean; and to be in that position means one will be nurse-handled. The attack in question time, when lecturing, has previously been connected with the battering and tearing of noise.

In my fantasies of lecturing, I always knew that the questions hurled at me would be fault-finding. Saying my lecture is no good is raising a stench; and the complicated language I expect in questioning is flinging faeces on my face (=the dirty-smelling flannel). To belittle what I have to say, by inferring that it has little or no importance, is "wet-blanketing" me; that is exposing my wet body to the cold air.

Also, questioning time after a lecture is the cleaning that takes place after baby has messed its nappy. After birth I am awakened only for two things: to change my nappy and for food. But as nappy changing takes place, even if I am awakened for food, it becomes a matter of *fact* that I suffer an attack *every time* I awake.

Soon after I started the shivering, while drawing last night, R.M. began to encourage me to continue and I said, pettishly, "I don't want to wake up. I want to sleep. It hurts".

Whenever I had decided to do some work in these last few days, either drawing or the compilation of the book, I found myself dropping with sleep.

To do something meant making a stool and, therefore, bringing me nearer to a nurse-attack; so, it was safer for me to get to sleep.

On going to bed after this last set of drawings I found that my hot-water-bottle had been forgotten. I became aware of this before sleeping and wondered if I should get up and get one. I then thought, "I might get some new light on my need for the bottle if I try to do without it". As a consequence, I slept very lightly; being only half asleep. My mind was still at work in this semi-conscious state. Although some dream was in progress my conscious mind was carrying on at the same time. I thought, "The bottle is the breast, (it had come up previously as that). But why can't I sleep without it?" And then the answer came: "The breast as breast is not the reason why you want it. It is being with mother in bed; and you are saying that 'it is only when I am with mother in bed that I am safe from nurse' ".

Thus, I can only sleep and be awake in safety while in mother's bed because mother never attacks. It is only when the nurse comes and takes me away from mother that I am attacked.

I can understand now that my intolerance of dirt in almost any form has been due to my unconscious fear and knowledge that if I am contaminated with dirt I shall be attacked.

A sloppy bit of work or thinking, or anything not well done and brought to a clean finish, is dangerous. Any untidiness, which, in the process of daily life must happen in relation to so many things, such as one's papers, cupboards, work and so on, fill me with a kind of despair. I feel overwhelmed and find the greatest difficulty in tidying anything up that has become untidy. There is what almost amounts to a feeling of sickness at the time I contemplate having to tidy up. The feeling is due to the recognition that what has happened is symbolically a wetting and dirtying of my nappy and that now I shall be attacked by the nurse.

The indications that assimilation had taken place came that afternoon and evening. I was again aware that my taste had resumed the normal for I was enjoying my food and remarked to that effect at table. Also, I am not feeling cold so much and I lay down on the couch today without being covered with a rug and having the electric fire on, even though it is considerably colder today than it has been. This afternoon while out in the car I began singing again after an interval of several months and I behaved with complete freedom and jollity, which is an indication with me of the reduction of fear. I am altogether more awake today.

This finishes the material I am presenting to you today. It is two months or more since this occurred. Since then, I have had no further fears of death which, previously, had been a nightly nightmare to me. Immediately following this piece of analysis, I tidied all my drawers and many untidy corners about the house. I have had no further body twitching which had come on during analysis and increased up to this point. And, finally, I was able for the first time to sit down to do the work of this demonstration and carry it through to a finish. Previously, anxiety would commence the moment I settled down to it and after an hour or so would be too great for me to carry on.

And now to close this paper with a brief summing up. I hope that in what I have shown you I shall have proved my claims, namely, that the pace of emergence into consciousness of unconscious material has been increased and that the thoroughness with which it is done is more complete than by the usual method. With regard to the therapeutic result, I feel that has been evident this evening to some of those present. I came to psycho-analysis originally as a so-called normal person. I needed it for professional purposes. Previous to analysis I had been a remarkably efficient and successful woman in all my undertakings. After seven years analysis my physical health collapsed under the strain. Psychologically I was left battered and broken. I had no strength left in me to carry on. When I first came to analysis, I told my analyst that the only signs I could trace in myself as evidence of neurosis were, (1) that I had a distant, faint fear of death and; (2) that I had never been able to speak in public except under the most pressing circumstances and that then I would far rather be shot than have to do it.

I no longer have any haunting fear of death. I have given this evening's demonstration without the slightest rise in my pulse rate, whereas previously I should have been unable to voice my opinions to any group of fellow analysts.

It is because some of you have known me before that I have chosen myself as the "rabbit" for this evening's demonstration.

Note

1 This lecture was given in 1938. There is no information on where it was held and who the members of the audience were.

Chapter 4

The scientific aspect of Surrealism[1]

SURREALISM is one of the outcomes of a demand, on the part of those dissatisfied with the world, for the complete liberation of mankind from all fetters which prevent full expression. Humankind demands full expression. It is a biological necessity.

In 1934 André Breton, one of the founders of Surrealism and its present leader, defined Surrealism as:

> Pure psychic automatism, by which it is intended to express, verbally in writing or by other means, the real *process* of thoughts. Thought's dictation in the absence of all control exercised by the reason and outside all aesthetic or moral preoccupations.
>
> (p. 59, italics added)

Psycho-analysis, although originally the outcome of a different aim, also strives to free the psychology of the individual from internal conflict so that she or he may function freely. Thus it can be assumed that the final goal of Surrealism and Psycho-analysis is the same—the liberation of man—but that the approach to this end is by different paths.

During the process of a research, undertaken from the psycho-analytic point of view (by my colleague and myself), the results of certain experiments in painting and drawing led to Surrealism. A considerable amount of interesting material was collected and in it some of the real values of Surrealism became manifest. As a detailed description of the progress of this research is impossible in the limited space of this journal only a brief idea of some of the results, and the light these throw on the whole subject of art, will be practicable.

It is well-known that unconscious fantasy is at work in all Surrealist creations; but that the fantasy-story the unconscious is unfolding is intelligible is not such common knowledge. The telling of some of those stories is one of the purposes of this article. Although the method by which the interpretations of drawings and paintings were obtained is complicated the results are crystal-clear. For instance it can be clearly demonstrated that one

DOI: 10.4324/9781003333098-4

unconscious meaning of traditional art (art that has become established and accepted) is painting according to parental wishes, or to please the parent. Such creations may display excellent craftsmanship but very little, if any, of the creator's basic personality, and vitality is restricted.

Further, it is possible to show that painting freely, that is Surrealistically, may, in the unconscious, mean either the making of a mess, a diarrhoea or a preference for making stools all over the place instead of into the chamber. On the other hand it may have quite opposite meanings as, for example, the making of a child, or the search for something of interest in the stools. But whatever the act of painting may symbolise there is always an underlying reason for it. A fantasy is in progress and a story is being told, as the following example and interpretation illustrate.

This drawing of a man having his eye gouged out has in it the wish to get into the father to find a safe place from an unsafe external world. The reason for the need for flight is also stated in this picture. The man's tongue is torn by his own teeth, in disapproval of himself. The drawing is expressing fear of the man who would do such a thing to himself as punishment for his own

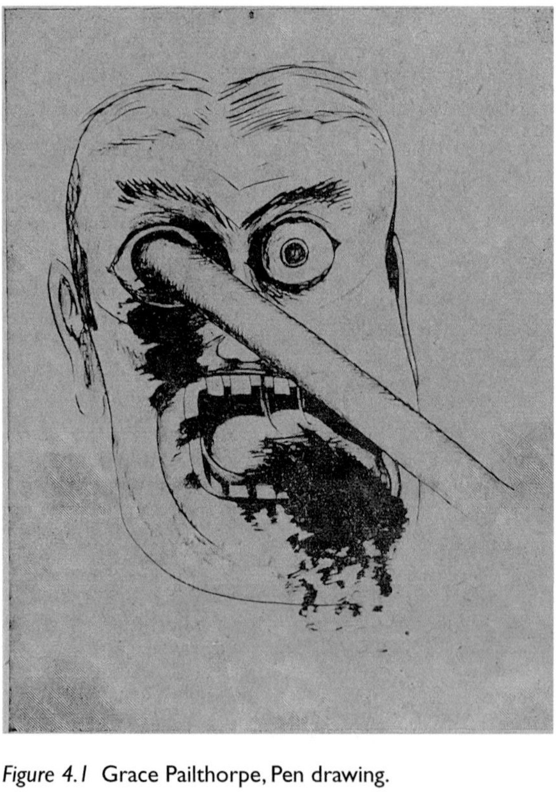

Figure 4.1 Grace Pailthorpe, Pen drawing.

misdoings, and 'If,' it is argued, 'this is what he does to himself for his bad behaviour, what would he do to me if he caught me wanting to behave badly? I must find a good way to escape his anger.' And so a hole is bored into the man and a hideout is found in his body. The act portrayed by the infantile unconscious, about which this fear had arisen, was that of stealing milk from the mother.

In this research material there is evidence of the fact that early enforced restrictions on the infant's excretory functions inhibits fantasy life and, therefore, its imagination. A healthy or balanced imagination is of vital importance. The repression, of this faculty, which lack of understanding has made widespread, leads to a condition which the New Testament describes as, 'a house divided against itself which cannot stand'. Thus today there is the slow disintegration of all civilizations because the units that constitute society are not psychologically (and, therefore, not biologically) integrated.

Art within the confines of any tradition is like an animal in a cage. An imprisoned creature will lose much of its inherent grandeur and vitality. A cramped freedom can only permit a mockery of life. There is little scope for fantasy within the cage of tradition-bound art. Art that is free from restriction becomes alive, colourful and vital.

When, however, such barriers to freedom are symbolically destroyed by an act of will and a Surrealist career begun, the discovery that movement is still difficult is soon made. So early endeavours in Surrealist art often are, to trained eyes, lacking in the essential qualities. This is due to the fact that firmly established inhibitions still maintain their hold no matter how much self-permission to be free is given. This is one reason why some give up their efforts, complaining that Surrealism leads nowhere. But Surrealism can lead to a greater understanding of the world around and within us, and it is a matter of time only before this will be recognised. It is impossible to create a well-organised external world *unless at the same time* the internal mental world is harmonised, since it is only through mental acquiescence on the part of the units that go to form the whole machinery of civilization that it can function smoothly. Further, the understanding of the world around us is reached by means of our sense organs and if these are not functioning freely we are not capable of getting an accurate focus upon the happenings that affect us.

With these preliminary remarks in mind we can now turn to the consideration of some selected paintings and drawings.

'Free translations' from the works of some of our prominent Surrealist painters, such as Dali, Miro or Tanguy, may be interesting but they would be unreliable. They would be entertaining but they would not fit into the purpose of this article. Concrete facts are more convincing and, for this reason, the examples given are taken from the research since, in this case, one can answer for the accuracy of the interpretations.

Before giving the interpretations of the following illustrations it is necessary to impress upon the mind that *the infantile fantasies underlying the pictures are not in consciousness at the time of painting or drawing*. The unconscious story is brought into consciousness by a special technique. Thus a hill or a house mean exactly what they are to the artist while working. All that is known at the time is that a house is appearing, a hill is appearing, and so on. To the degree that one is able to give oneself entirely up to the dictates of the unconscious, to that degree the perfect story will be told. Conscious interference in the painting can always be detected, since it invariably distorts the story in the fantasy-creation.

This fantasy picture is of the artist himself. He is depicted as having an animal head with a huge mouth. On top of his head is a cock's-comb; and under the lower jaw is a dark, beard-like arrangement of wavy lines. From his mouth proceed smudges and feather-like shapes. On his leg is an inverted flower-shape from which some drops are falling. Under this, lying in a wooden box, is the shape of a dead bird.

The underlying unconscious fantasy is that the artist has killed his mother and is now enjoying himself with playing with the mess the kill has provided for him. To do this he has first to decorate himself with a cock's-conb and the beard. By doing this he is putting himself into the position of *those who are permitted to kill*. In his childhood he has witnessed 'kosher-killing' of poultry. Priests with beards become to his child-mind the *people*

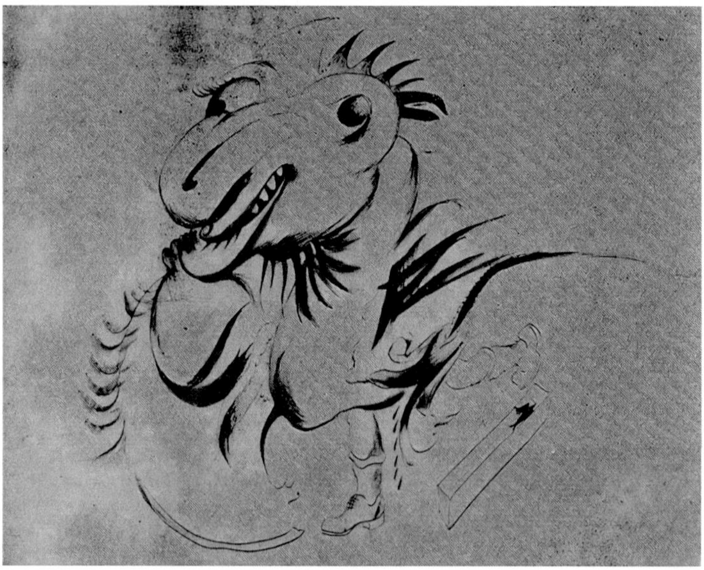

Figure 4.2 Reuben Mednikoff, *Come Back Soon*.

who may kill; therefore, in his fantasy, he first makes himself into a priest with a beard. To make doubly sure he is this kind of a priest and none other he puts the cock's-comb on his head. Thus he is saying, 'I am a priest who kills chicken'. It may not be generally known that this form of killing birds and animals for the table is a religious rite and is only performed by those set aside for this purpose. The dead bird represents the mother. The title which the artist gave to this drawing was 'Come back soon'. Death as an extinction of life does not exist in the realm of the unconscious. So although the play of the moment demands the death of the mother in order to play with the mess, he makes sure of its impermanence by his title. The inverted flower represents the fowls he had seen hung up upside-down from which blood dripped. It is not necessary to go into further details as to the fuller meaning of the picture. It suffices to demonstrate the importance of every detail of the picture. It will be noted that even the character of the lines is of importance. The smudgy quality of those lines symbolise the nature of his play while the drop-like character of that which in the flower are the stamens, are a further example of it.

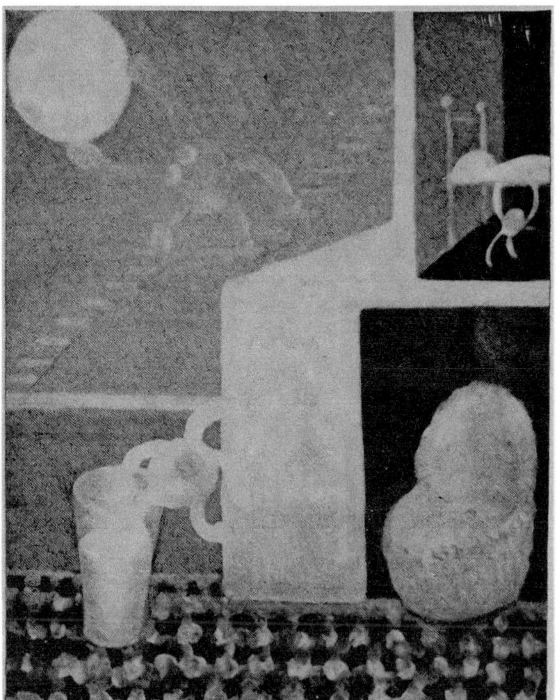

Figure 4.3 Grace Pailthorpe, *Oil, April I* (1938).

Here the unconscious fantasy is simple. The artist is represented as a baby in a cot, asleep. The rest of the painting is what the baby is dreaming. It sends forth its hand—the little animal with five limbs (five fingers)—on a journey. It first seeks the sun, a symbol of the breast, getting there by climbing stairs. This is the groping of the baby's hand towards the mother's breast while in her lap. The next scene, in the top right corner, is the baby-hand climbing into the mother-bed, the other place where it has experienced feeding. The third effort is to get milk from a glass of milk near-by, to the left of the cot. The picture is therefore saying, 'I wish to be fed. I must find that breast that feeds me'. The position of the cot, which is half in and half out of a room, is the position of a pram on a verandah and conveys the idea of a sleep in the day-time. The need of the moment in the artist's life brings up the wish-fantasy to be back in the infantile situation when sleep and feeding merged blissfully into one, and where wishes were quickly fulfilled.

This unconscious fantasy-picture depicts the artist as a child running behind a house. The house is a symbol of mother. He has stolen the ball, a breast symbol, and the father tree is after him to punish him for this theft. The branch projecting from the tree in the direction of the ball is the father's hand stretching forward to feel the breast-ball to see if he, the child, has damaged it. The steps behind the child are one way of escape. The hill is the mother's skirt. He can run round behind her and dodge father this way, a thing the artist frequently did as a child when trying to escape the father's wrath and punishment. But the child in the painting is running to get to the ladder

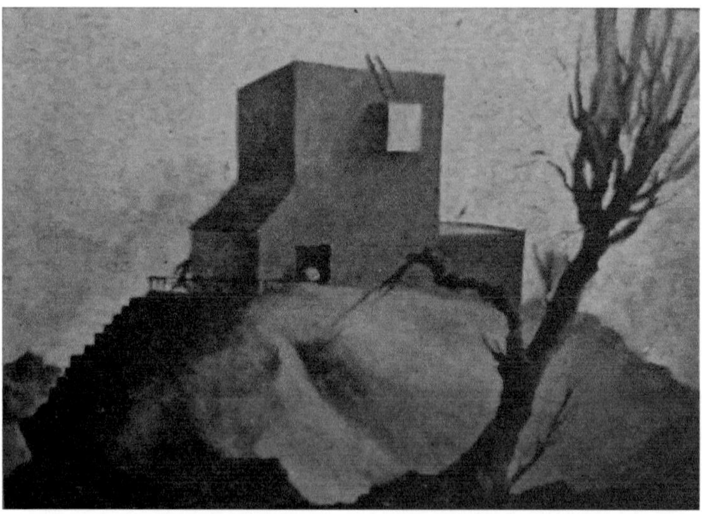

Figure 4.4 Reuben Mednikoff, *Oil, September 19* (1935).

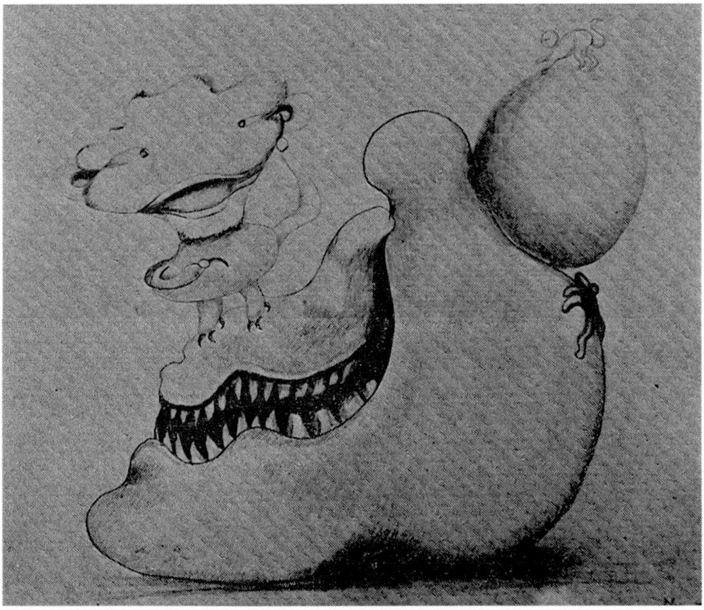

Figure 4.5 Grace Pailthorpe, *Pencil drawing* (1938).

and so on to the roof. The roof is the mother's head. In other words, a child is safe only when it is high up in the mother's arms, where it is level with the mother's head. There were further details in this painting but enough has been given in demonstration of the story being told.

This again depicts a simple, direct unconscious wish-fantasy. The little figure standing on a jaw-bone represents the artist. It has a claw finger on each hand with which it can scratch. It is pointing to its ear and to its belly to indicate where it wants to scratch. The jaw it is standing on is the mother's face. The small figure climbing up behind the jaw is again the same little person and so too is the monkey on the ball shape above. This ball represents the mother's head and the back of the jaw the mother's shoulder. The picture is saying, 'I have two irritating places for which I can get no relief except in being held close to the mother's head, neck and shoulder'.

All these pictures came into being as a result of the experimental work of the research.

The details and interpretations of these pictures have necessarily been curtailed; but they serve to show the quantity of interest held within the bounds of each. Not a line or detail is out of place and everything has its symbolic meaning. This also applies to colour. Every mark, shape and colour is *intended*, by the unconscious and has its meaning.

The unconscious is a master in its own form of art and its creations have qualities similar to those demanded of any form of art, whatever the media. It tells its story perfectly; with economy of language and with associations that convey the maximum effect. It gives only those details necessary for the complete understanding of its moods. It tells a perfect short story. Simplicity, directness and lucidity are its aims. It conforms to all that has vitality, perfection of rhythm and composition—and it cannot be ignored because it is truth expressed with vitality.

Perhaps these statements seem an exaggeration, but to be aware of the complete story, which it has been impossible to give in this limited space, would be to dispel any doubts.

Every unconscious creation is not a work of art but where complete freedom has been possible the results are perfect in balance, design, colour, rhythm and possess a vitality that is not to be found anywhere else than in Surrealism. Because it is free from the limitations of traditionalism its movements have greater variation and infinitely greater daring.

Unfortunately such paintings and drawings create a feeling of fear or distaste on the part of the public; but if they can bring themselves to look again and again they begin to feel an inexplicable attraction towards these pictures. They are being drawn towards a freedom which they, too, would like to experience. Eventually they admit that, although they do not understand Surrealism, there is an indefinable attraction which excites them. And many artists, who still conform to the dictates of traditionalism, have admitted to being profoundly affected by the vitality of the colour, movement and design of Surrealist creations.

At present we are in the early stages of this form of art. The infantile unconscious can only become free gradually. Its stiffened limbs have to overcome the effects of previous binding. It has to overcome the fear of abandoning its cage, which is in large part of its own making in protection of itself from attacks from the external world. Until these bonds are broken and 'limbs' are fully stretched it will be impossible to get that perfection which is called 'creation'—the conglomeration of qualities that make a thing 'live', and by which it stands the test of time.

We are witnesses of the birth of a new form of art, of the transitional period during its progress from within to without. Surrealism is ushering into the world an art greater than has hitherto been known, for its potentialities are limitless. And this art of the future will arrive when completely freed fantasy evolves from uninhibited minds. It will be the dawn of a new art epoch.

As long as fantasy-life, or the imaginative life, is free it learns by experience. The fantasies produced are richer in quality and content as a result of experience. But fantasy or imagination bound by early infantile inhibitions and fears remains infantile in what it creates. In the process of becoming free Surrealist paintings, drawings and sculpture will necessarily be infantile in content. This does not preclude its right to be called art. The infantile fantasy, as it becomes freer and experiences more as a result of that freedom, will grow increasingly more adult in character and its creations will show it.

Imagination travels well in harness with reason. The infant human comes into the world with a remarkable power to reason. It reasons through its senses. Its mistakes are not through lack of power to reason but through lack of experience. Hitherto humanity has stressed the value of reason and has restricted imagination. Imagination and reason are biological twins.

They must grow up together. What affects the one will affect the other. If their development is such that one grows apace and the other remains stunted the results are disastrous. The growth of our imagination and reason must, like our mental and physical development, be balanced. They are interdependent. The crippling of one or other has its immediate effect on the living organism. The inhibition of fantasy-life, from whatever cause (internal or external), must result in a crippled creation. Equally, any loss of freedom in the use of one's reason results in a similar distortion. According to the degree we suffer from such mishandling, to that degree we are narrow, hidebound, mentally unhappy and limited individuals and, at worst, are among the many unfortunates who end their days in asylums, workhouses or prisons.

Surrealism is a serious project. If followed wholeheartedly to its final goal it has the power to bring happiness to all humanity. But it is a discipline, and one that must be persistently pursued if anything of value is to be the outcome and if disaster is to be avoided. There are no half-way houses. There are many dangers in the achievement of this aim but these can be circumnavigated. The object of Surrealism is to know the self. All the sages of the past have advocated self-knowledge but they have not shown us how to reach that ideal. Here is the opportunity.

Note

1 This article was first published in the *London Bulletin* (1938–39, 7:10–16).

Chapter 5

Primary processes of the infantile mind demonstrated through the analysis of a prose-poem[1]

Before putting forward the details of the analysis of the prose-poem, and the conclusions that resulted therefrom, I present the poem.

REINCARNATION

The world was dark … black and dusty sepia with crawling green and livid putrefaction. Not a soul was about. The noiseless creep of the maggoty mobs moved from glut to glut. A flutter of wind made the noisome stench rise and hit savagely at nostrils which were not there. Nothing was there but hideous, cruel nothingness maniacally slashing this way and that; torturing itself to reach and crush a human sense.

And then it came. Out of that putrescent mass a seethe and slump, slow rising, slow sinking. And the air stood stiller, held petrified lest what it sought had come.

The stilled and overpowering stench closed up ready for its lethal spring.

The seethe appeared once more, took shape as an 'excrescing' pimple, black-green with poisonous maroon purplings, and venous-blooded specks flirted with orange slits.

In hysterical rage lest death should rise again, the concentrated stench flung itself upon the offending seethe. And down it flumped, splayed out like a liquid mud, into the sucking mass.

But life was there, a flicker so small it only felt itself as there against the thing that pressed upon it; and in that knowledge was the last thread broken.

From out that liqufeying lump shot forth the foulest miscenations and grappling with the great flat lumping hand that held it down bit and tore it to shreds.

This done, it rose on all fours, struggled drunkenly its unplanned course, knowing there was a confine to the clammy, noisome world which held it. From out that confine it would hurl itself or, failing, know no more.

At last the goal was reached. Stripping the slime-weighted garments away from her stricken body—tearing away with teeth and nails a piece

DOI: 10.4324/9781003333098-5

here, a piece there—at last she stood naked and torn at the edge of the murky, mud-bubbling cauldron that had held her. Frantically she flung herself from off the edge into bottomless space. For oeons in that blank was held, and drifted in unconscious ecstasy in primal rhythm.

* * *

The oeons passed and once again that naked body made movement, so slight it hardly could be felt—and once again the nothingness was roused to express itself against intruding life. The battle now was lightly played, and puff and duff, and flut and plut, and scuff and scut, the bodies squirling in and out each other.

And suddenly she was there—solid, full-formed, sitting on a stool. Arm uplifted. All brightness was around her. The light and blue and coolth of bubbling life once more filled her suffocating lungs.

Her uplifted arm worked swiftly and no breathless sound intruded. Out on that canvas she poured her life in one immortal ecstasy. Her life was done. She slept. An oeon passed of sweet dreamless drift before she woke again.

In presenting the analysis of the prose-poem 'Reincarnation' I have two specific objects in view:

1. To demonstrate the *process of thought* in the infant and so to understand the details of sensation and experience that go to produce the early steps in reasoning. Thought processes are at work at birth but consciousness of them as such is, of course, absent. This came out clearly in the re-experiencing of birth-traumata by the writer of the poem during analysis.
2. To show that when the unconscious has *free* action in inspiring poetry, or prose poetry, no phrase or word is superfluous in the word picture that is drawn. The infantile unconscious practices, instinctively, that economy of language, that directness and simplicity in style that is inherent in good literature. The subject matter may not appeal to the reader or listener and the reading of it may induce an unpleasant emotion; but, in either case, there is no denying the strength and vitality of the emotion expressed. The mode of expression may be new. It may function outside the limits set by traditionalists; nevertheless it is impossible to get away from the above-mentioned qualities with regard to it.

The author of this prose-poem felt, as it emerged, that it was depicting reincarnation. Reincarnation is the theory which she finds the most acceptable of all religious beliefs. In this myth we have the opportunity of enjoying life in gradation. As experience grows the individual is able to enjoy a greater and ever-increasing richness in the act of living. But this ideal is futile until release from the original psychological traumata of previous lives has been accomplished.

The prose-poem is in two sections. It gives the brief story of two awakenings into life—two reincarnations. In the first there is little sense of self-consciousness. Consciousness is only of the external consciousness—the 'not-me' awareness. Self-consciousness can come only through free expression. Thus, in the first section, because external or 'not-me' consciousness is of a distressing nature the birth of the world (or individual) is entirely unpleasant. When the unpleasantness is at last removed the world (or unit) once more goes into æonic oblivion. In the second birth self-consciousness appears and with it self-expression. Because of self-consciousness the opportunity for self-expression is there and is immediately seized. Life's rhythm runs its normal course—birth, expression and sleep. The cycle repeats itself.

In analysing a poem, or any work of art, we know that there are two aspects, or levels, from which it may be viewed: from the reality or conscious aspect and from the unconscious. The reality situation here is that the author felt herself to be portraying a conception of the birth of a world, and all there was therein—the greater including the less. She felt it applied, equally, to the universe, a planet, an animal or an insect; in fact to all life whatever its form.

From the unconscious layer, analysis gradually revealed the specific meaning of the poem in relation to the infantile unconscious o the writer. While accepting for the moment the author's theories that the microcosm is a replica of the macrocosm in all its biological qualities, one was able, step by step, to reach the unconscious meaning of every phrase of the poem. Because of lack of space it must be given in a compressed form. I shall give a direct translation, adding explanatory notes only where it is felt to be advisable.

The scene is a cradle. A new-born babe is in it.

'*The world was dark* ...' indicates it is night. '... *black and dusty sepia* ...' refers to the colour sensation of darkness. '... *with crawling green and livid putrefaction*.' Here the reference is to the crawling sensation of gases within the bowels and the colour-impression '*green and livid*' was due to eye sensations caused by the congestion from held-in breath. '*Putrefaction*' denotes a general noisome smell of enclosed body and napkin aromas. It is a picture of that darkness and its accompaniments and all it meant in sensation to the infant, run into one sentence.

'*Not a soul was about*.' This means everything was absolutely quiet. There was no other life or movement within that room.

'*The noiseless creep of the maggoty mobs moved from glut to glut*.' This is conveying the sensation of the gaseous movement of the bowels; first in one part of the abdomen and then in another.

Note

1 This article was first published in the *International Journal of Psycho-Analysis* (1941, 22:44–59).

Chapter 6

Deflection of energy, as a result of birth trauma, and its bearing upon character formation[1]

In this paper I shall demonstrate, through the analysis of a patient, how the whole quantum of energy of a new-born infant comes to be regulated and controlled; and the bearing of a carefully reasoned disposal of this energy, by the infant, upon the character in adult life.

The patient in question was a young man. He was capable, successful in his work, and with great latent ability which, however, he felt he was not using or able to use to capacity. He had certain character difficulties.

An early marriage had been unsuccessful and the parties had eventually separated. It was soon after the divorce that he came for analysis. At that time he was in a physically run-down condition. He had been neglecting himself, and his general appearance was such that he looked almost twice his age.

It should be mentioned that I gave this patient a new form of psychoanalytic treatment in which various graphic media are used as a vehicle of expression. The technique cannot be given here as space forbids. As the material that follows will convey, even though given in tabloid form, it brings up unconscious fantasy much more readily and with a far greater presentation of detail than by the classic method. The whole of the material of this section of the patient's analysis, including the birth trauma which is only touched upon here, covered a period of one month and five days.

An infant is born in possession of great vitality. Of what magnitude it is in relation to its weight and size, I do not know, but the manifestations of it are instantly visible, audible and tactile to everyone who has to deal with the newborn. The vocal power of the infant is phenomenal when it is considered that a few moments before birth the respiratory apparatus had never functioned. Its arms and legs move with remarkable rapidity and strength. Its power to micturate and defecate are immediately set in motion, both during and after birth. One cannot but wonder at the miracle of change that has been wrought. A few hours ago the fetus was lying quiescent, or almost so, in the womb and, within a short while, it is transformed into a little mass of loudly protesting humanity, full of a vast quantity of vitality of limb and lung.

DOI: 10.4324/9781003333098-6

Could we go through life with that initial vitality at our disposal, what would be the result? By the time we are full grown and settled to a way of life, how much of that original measure of vigor is left us, to do with it what we will? It is of the essential vitality with which we are born that this paper will deal.

To introduce the subject of the disposal of energy it is necessary briefly to narrate the experiences of the infant in the prenatal stage just prior to and during birth.

From the fifth month a fetus begins to move. Movements can be vigorous or feeble, frequent or infrequent, from that time onward. There comes a moment, however, when the uterus resents the size and movements of the fetus and commences to respond by contractions. As the unborn child grows to maturity it becomes, by reason of its size, more restricted in its movement. Contractions of the uterus begin to turn it into a position ready for ejection, usually head downward.

It was apparent from the analysis of the patient, whose case material I use to illustrate this article, that he had, while still in utero, resented the discomfort of the occipital position, and had 'kicked himself back' into the previous position. This activity was repeated again and again, until the contractions had become too strong for the fetus and made it impossible for it to resume the original position. The act of birth, that is of being forcibly expelled from the womb, was thought by the infant to be a punishment for its kicking. The numerous other pains and hurts also, that it suffered at and immediately after birth, were thought to be additional punishment for the initial kicking. In the extremity of compulsion it wished heartily to destroy that which was compressing and extruding it.

The baby developed, even at this early stage, a strong idea that, if it became angry and resisted aggressively it always was punished for it; for whenever it suffered discomfort and started energetic kicking, arm flailing and screaming it found itself 'attacked'. The attentions of the mother, or nurse, to its bodily needs was thought to be chastisement for its violent activity and aggressive hate towards what it felt was interfering with it. In addition to its muscular and vocal aggression it had defecated in anger during the process of birth, and this act, too, was felt to be revenged by the expulsion from the uterus. The fetus had defecated in a paroxysm of hate of the relentless attack on its body which was forcing it onward against its will. Muscular movement and hate became interlocked. It wished to destroy the womb. The pains and shocks that immediately followed birth were, so it thought, punishment for its wishes to destroy.

A vicious circle was set up. When it was attacked it tried to destroy, and then it was punished, that is attacked again, and so must destroy again; and thus the infant came to 'know' that punishment would follow every angry use of its body against interference.

After the cataclysmic rat-a-tat of the birth traumata was over sleep from exhaustion followed. When the baby woke it was uncomfortable and began to cry and to struggle once more. Instantly the nurse's hands and fingers, which were painful to the child's sensitive body, began a series of 'attacks'; and once again it screamed and kicked in anger. As its cries were not followed by an immediate cessation of the handling to which it was being subjected, it imagined that its sufferings were being inflicted in retaliation for its angry fighting against the attacking hands.

In the case of this patient, however, energy was not used solely to combat repetitive 'attacks' upon him. It was used also to control his instinctive responses. 'If my kicking and anger at being thwarted or hurt is attacked by further pain, then', reasoned the infant—and how sound the reasoning was had the premises been correct, 'there is only one thing left for me to do, and that is to restrain my kicking and my anger'. But even so, although kicking was subdued to a minimum, and the baby's other activities also, the discomforture and hurts came with each awakening. Napkin changing, which involved a number of uncomfortable buffetings, occurred each time it awoke from sleep, either of its own accord or by being lifted up by the nurse. Frantically it searched its mind and experience, limited as then it was, to find a means of warding off these ever recurring assaults.

Restraint, applied to the point of strain, became the rule in relation to any of its instinctual habits which were felt to be the cause of punishment. The strength of the inhibitive force needed to bring about the curbing of its normal impulses naturally used up much of the infant's vitality. On finding that even by such measures it could not control the situation, fear of its complete helplessness caused still further consumption of energy. The feeling of utter helplessness was too great to be endured and, as a consequence, a major part of its energy had to be deflected from the main stream to deal with the situation.

In order to show exactly how deflection takes place, I will recount, in some detail, some of the specific sufferings this patient experienced at birth. Although it is the story of one person's birth agony, it will be recognized that most of what occurred to this infant befalls all infants, whatever differences there may be in the method adopted to deal with the situations against which they may have to contend. In reading what follows it is necessary to remember that the major necessity of an infant is to control its surroundings.

It has already been told how the fetus had kicked and defecated in utero and how its ejection was thought to be revenge against its aggressiveness. The next infliction of pain followed quickly. The child's buttocks were slapped, causing it to scream and to kick and flail its arms vigorously to 'throw off' the hurt that had assailed it. At the same time a sharp pain at the cut end of the umbilicus was felt and it seemed to the infant as if the buttock slapping had pushed the pain through to that point. This additional torture was too much and, in its fury and agony of protest, it was seized with an uncontrollable paroxysm of muscular convulsion. The experience of the body itself being thrown into this overwhelming and uncontrollable state was terrifying. The paroxysm continued until complete exhaustion was reached—another appalling experience. Each fresh suffering was imagined to be the punishment for the original attack upon the uterus. It had wished to destroy the womb utterly. Thus, it was being destroyed utterly in return. The experience, so annihilating to the baby, was felt as a destructive assault in retaliation. Its exhausted condition, and the fact that the pain remained in spite of all its efforts to disperse it, forced upon it the realization of its utter helplessness. Added to the recognition that it could not control pain by trying to 'throw it off' was the realization that it dare not even attempt to do so, for such an effort brought additional punishment—the pain of its whole body being shaken helplessly to a state of complete and final exhaustion. Terror of a repetition of such a crisis forced it to build up defenses against any possible renewal of such an overwhelming of its whole being. From that moment it learned to resist the expression of its instinctive impulses to meet attack with attack, and, for this purpose, a large amount of energy was deflected and shut off from the main stream. This was not the end. Another painful experience was about to happen which would add still further to the necessity of curbing natural responses.

When partially recovered from the semi-unconscious state to which exhaustion had brought it, the infant once again felt the pain at its umbilicus and began weakly to cry and kick. This activity initiated a pain in its head, described by the patient as a 'hot head' and an 'aching head'. It was yet another penalty for protesting and trying to 'throw off' pain.

At this point an interesting assessment of the use made of its energy took place in the infant's mind. Muscular paroxysm and exhaustion was felt to be a punishment for using the whole power of its body in repelling 'pain. A 'hot and aching head' (due to its strained effort when exhausted) was felt to be the penalty for using 'the last drop of energy' in striving to rid itself of pain. Thus its dynamic vitality had been divided into two quantities of force. With the establishment of this idea the use of its energy was controlled by the consideration of these two quantities. Therefore, in order to avoid a recurrence of these terrifying experiences, it curtailed the expenditure of its energy and doled it out in such a way as to evade, first, the use of energy with every ounce of strength behind it; and second, the use of the last fraction of energy. For safety it had to keep well within these two extremes.

As a consequence of this early conditioning, the patient, in adult life, was unable satisfactorily to apply himself to anything he undertook, unless the task was of short duration and did not require sustained effort. In other words, the best of his ability could be applied only in the case of a small task. A lengthy job would quickly arouse anxiety and his head would become 'hot and aching'. Also, any labor that demanded an all-out effort immediately brought on tiredness. This tiredness acted as a warning. On the slightest feeling of weariness he would instantly collapse. He would no longer be able to continue the work he was engaged upon. The physical tiredness was an indication that he was bringing himself to a state dangerously near the perilous moment of exhaustion. Any further effort beyond the point of feeling tired was hazardous, for it would mean he was employing all his energy. It became his habit to relax instantly he became aware of the slightest fatigue. He usually relapsed into an easy chair. Once he was settled comfortably it was virtually impossible for him to get up again, even if he needed to get something, until he was completely rested. This remarkable inertia persisted until all sign of fatigue had vanished since it served to check him from using his 'last drop of energy'. So, throughout life, after a short spell of work it became necessary for him to relax; or, if circumstances compelled him to continue he would begin to seek another and less arduous job. No employment must be allowed to bring him to a state of exhaustion, nor force him to use all his energy.

These restrictions in the use of energy affected him in other ways. He not only could not use his physical powers in the healthy adult way, but he had to avoid situations which would or were likely to put him into an equivocal position; that is, situations which might place him in a position of danger following the use of his energy. He was tolerant to a degree which was unnatural. He would never get angry. He avoided asserting himself, and even would not demand his rights lest he should precipitate an 'attack'. He did not wish to have to protest or to insist on his claims. He preferred to do without rather than to chance making an effort. In other words, he chose to avoid any form of aggressiveness since that implied the use of energy in attack. Yet, on the other hand, he would assert himself vigorously to maintain or realize a position of security from attack.

His hobbies were not manual, nor did they involve the use of his strength. He read a great deal and constantly went to the cinema. Thus, in his free time, he put himself in a position where no attack could arise. Since he was overanxious to see that his body was not taxed in any way he chose his friends from among those who did not indulge in active pleasures. In no way did he allow himself to be brought to a state of tiredness, for that condition aroused his unconscious fears.

Energy, therefore, as we have seen, had to be limited in expression. Whereas unrestrained vitality was a source of danger, it now transpired that inhibited energy could also be dangerous. One of the manifestations of this danger was quickly to appear.

Four activities had to be checked to avoid the punishment of pain. These were the limiting of leg activity, of arm activity, of bowel action and lastly, of crying. It is with the act of crying that I am first going to deal. The infant's last feeble effort in crying had become associated with head-aching as its punishment. To restrain its cries, however, was a greater strain than withholding its kicking and arm flailing. Further, the strain of checking its cries was a hurt in itself. Every adult, who, as a consequence of extreme distress, has had this natural urge and has had to refuse it expression, will know how severe a pain can arise out of this restraint. The child experienced this pain and, as a result, there arose another need—the need to avoid the strain of holding back its cries. To do this it must keep clear of situations which will lead to its being hurt, since pain caused it to cry. Thus the fear of the pain of strain added to the necessity of restraining its activities, its aggressive acts. Obviously during infancy contacts could not be avoided, therefore it was forced to cry and scream again and again. Avoidance of crying, however, was the infant's aim, even if circumstances made it impossible for it to succeed in its object. And so again, in adult life, shunning contacts with an outside world became imperative, and the repressed aim remained active. Rather than ask for something, when there was a doubt as to whether his demand would bring an angry refusal, he would not 'bother'. 'Why bother to do anything that will bring on upset (crying)' was a frequent saying of his. Doing without had become his method of evading uncertain issues. This attitude was an obstacle to all projects that might entail difficulties to be overcome, even when the ultimate purpose was pleasure. He had never wanted to risk a situation in which the slightest 'hurt' could be the outcome and thus many pleasures in life were foregone.

In the first few days of an infant's life so many things of a distressing and often painful nature impinge, in rapid succession, upon its person that one is compelled to wonder how it survives the trial. The infant, whose history we are following, had an even more devastating experience in store for it than any yet mentioned. It was more overwhelming in results than had been the multiple traumata of birth. Within a few days of its arrival into the world the baby was circumcised. At the moment immediately prior to the cutting of the foreskin its organ had been fingered and it gave the natural response to the handling. It urinated. Almost within the same instant, as it seemed to the infant, the severe and agonizing pain of the cut followed. This was an appalling 'punishment' for urinating. Nor was this the end. For days afterwards, at least seven or eight times a day (or more), each time it was compelled by nature to micturate it was 'punished' with the agony of acid on a wound. Suppression of the need to empty its bladder became a tormenting necessity. Once again the strain of withholding a function brought on pain, this time an ache in the testes. A difficult problem confronted it. Although leg activity can be controlled, urinating, like crying, or even more so than in the case of lachrymation, can never wholly be controlled.

What kind of a defense could the infant bring about to deal with this new predicament? The strain itself was the cause of the aching testes; but strain was necessary to control the flow of urine. Thus the defense against pain was itself painful. It now had to contend with the hurt it was experiencing at that precise moment, namely, the ache in the testes, and the fear of the acid pain that would immediately follow micturation. One of these would have to give way to the other. An existing pain is always a worse terror than a hurt not yet felt but only remembered, particularly if the pain being experienced reaches an intensity which is unbearable. To relieve the hurt of strain it gave way to its need to urinate, but only just so far as to relieve the tension which was the direct cause of the ache. It released only a small amount. As long as it did not make a forceful flow, that is completely empty its bladder, it felt safe from the other infliction, the cut; for it was the forceful ejection of urine, which took place when its penis was handled, that brought on this worst of all pains, so it thought. The soreness of the wound, revived by the acid trickle, was excruciating enough, but the other hurt was too shattering to risk any repetition of it. The severe smarting of the wound caused it to cry and this brought the mother to its side. She would apply a salve to the organ which eased the smart. As a result of the dressing of the wound the acid hurt was of short duration. Its mind began classifying its hurts. A short agonizing pain was preferable to the hurt of circumcision which was far greater in agony and appeared to last longer.

These defenses, viz., the holding up of urination to the last limit of tension, and then the release of a small quantity only at a time, were the best that it could devise. Suppression of the need to micturate, in order to avoid punishment, continued long after there ceased to be a necessity to do so. The threat of a repetition of the unbearable torment was relegated to the unconscious and with it the defense mechanisms to deal with the situation. That being so, we should expect to find traces of this early injury appearing in adulthood. This we do.

The analysand had never been able to be aware of his need to urinate until the very last moment when the necessity to do so would suddenly become violently imperative. This state of affairs had led to many awkward moments. This, however, was not the only aftermath of the situation. When he did relieve himself he could only do a little; and so in a short while he would need to micturate again. This would continue until, by a series of small quantities, he had completely emptied his bladder. Needless to say, the affliction was of considerable inconvenience in social life. Obviously the long repressed original necessity to relieve pressure and painful tension by a prescribed method of urination had continued throughout life.

It has been shown that the infant had avoided a forceful flow of its urine in dealing with its problem of evading strain. The reason why a forceful flow had to be avoided follows.

When, at the circumcision, the infant's penis had been handled it had urinated forcefully in pleasure. Ejection of fluid, as a result of titillation of the organ, is orgasmic in force and a complete evacuation of the bladder is effected. Because of the agony of the cut the unrestrained discharge of urine had to be curbed. With this curbing another form of natural expression became inhibited. The infant felt, very naturally, that his urinating was not liked, since the outcome was the cutting of its foreskin. Because it had urinated in pleasure, as a response to the titillation by the fingers of the operator, it assumed that the pleasure in the act of urination was forbidden. Thus it had now not only to defend itself against an unrestrained discharge of urine, but also against the taking of pleasure in the function itself. The result was that it inhibited its pleasure-feeling in its responses to titillation.

These two restraints were to react upon the patient throughout life. He was never able to show pleasure or forcefulness in any of his actions. When he was enjoying himself most his outward appearance was grave, and quite often more than grave, for his expression was frequently one of boredom. He is secretly enjoying pleasure but must not show that he is pleased. Until this part of his analysis was dealt with he had always been mystified by this characteristic. He had often wondered why, even though he was enjoying himself immensely, he could not give any visible indication of his pleasure.

The prohibition of the expression of pleasure-energy brought about a 'tiredness', the warning to cease activity which, in this case, was to hold back from taking pleasure. The locking-up of his energy in the expression of pleasure produced strain in his surroundings. The inhibitions interfered with his family relationships. He was gloomy and lacked enthusiasm and this was resented by his more lively brothers and sisters. His incapacity for sustained action made him a poor companion for more vigorous associates. The only pleasures he could continue to enjoy were reading and the cinema, and this was because these occupations, as previous analysis had shown, symbolized breast-feeding. He had reason to feel that he was safe from attack while at the breast for it was only while he was feeding there that he was secure from interruption or the likelihood of experiencing excruciating pain.

The withholding, or locking-up, of energy from the main stream did not end here; nor was suppression the fate of all the energy that was abstracted from the main stream. A great deal of his dynamic vitality was held in reserve for 'ammunition purposes'. Since lachrymation and micturation were disapproved of and severely punished (and it will be shown later that defecation also came within this category), then some of the energy that would otherwise have been spent in these acts could be reserved for occasions when the infant could be aggressive, in a hidden way, and so get its revenge with impunity. As it found the use of its energy in a direct fashion (used forcefully) barred, the baby circumvented the prohibition by applying it negatively in attack. There were many instances of this inverted use of energy to be found in the analysand's behavior and character. For example, in discussion he would talk his opponent down and give no opportunity for the other person to respond. This was a symbolic urination to smother his opponent. He never kept to the point of the discussion, ignoring all arguments that might be raised in opposition to his own. On other occasions, during ordinary conversation, he would not hear, or would ignore, what was being said to him. When the talk was about a subject he did not like he paid no attention or would begin to talk of something else. In this way he interfered with the other person's activity (pleasure in conversation) in the same way as he felt his had been. In a multitude of little ways, none of them gross on their own but, by their constancy, adding up to an appreciable aggregate, he would stall another person's pleasurable activity. When asked to do something he invariably did it badly, thus hurting indirectly. It was a compulsion of his to differ in opinion or wish, even when the subject proposed was to his liking.

I have shown the consequences to this infant of the trauma of circumcision, and the deflection of energy from the healthy channels that followed. I will now demonstrate another deflection of a quantity of energy, this time relating to anal activities. Chronologically, the traumata occasioning anal inhibitions happened prior to the circumcision, but I have given the circumcision trauma first place because, in my opinion, the injury both at the time and in subsequent results was more far reaching and detrimental to the character and physical well-being of the analysand.

During the birth process the infant had defecated in fury and hate at what was happening to it, and in its fury all its energy was used. The uterus, which hitherto had been everything that a kindly cradle should be, had started to attack it, so it felt, and, panic-stricken, it had begun to fight for its life. It had tried to destroy the womb. For this destructive motion it was punished by being thrust out into the cold and then in having its stomach hurt, 'banged'— which analysis showed to be the pain felt when the umbilical cord was severed. After this first assault on its person it was set aside in a blanket. This covering was uncomfortable and constricted its movements. It imagined that it had been transposed from one womb to another. Because its new womb caused it discomfort it wished to rid itself of it just as it had done the other. For on emergence from the uterus it thought it had succeeded in its efforts in destruction of the womb. It now made another motion in anger. Again the aggressive act was followed by assault, this time from many fingers that inflicted innumerable little hurts. The handling of a new-born child is painful to a skin and the underlying muscles which hitherto have experienced nothing harsher than amniotic fluid. It was bathed and dressed. The cold, the unpleasant tasting water and the being moved and turned first this way and then that, caused acute suffering. To the infant it was all part of the chastisement. Finally, it is bound tightly in a binder which, because of its sore and throbbing cord, was extremely painful. Thus it is again hurt, 'banged', in the stomach for having defecated in anger. (It is impossible here to go extensively into detail, but every item of discomfort and pain during this process was brought up in rapid succession in analysis.) Even then painful experiences were not at an end. It soon discovered that every time it made a motion it was 'attacked' in a similar fashion, that is, made to suffer the discomforts of being cleaned and having its stomach 'banged' anew. The repetition of events made the infant feel, more than ever, that its motion was something that was not liked and that it was essential to restrain this act in the future. Once again energy had to be commandeered from the main flow to be used in withholding the physiological impulse to defecate when the occasion arrived.

Still further details, however, were brought to light. Since the infant could no more control its motions absolutely than it could because, in my opinion, the injury both at the time and in subsequent results was more far reaching and detrimental to the character and physical well-being of the analysand.

During the birth process the infant had defecated in fury and hate at what was happening to it, and in its fury all its energy was used. The uterus, which hitherto had been everything that a kindly cradle should be, had started to attack it, so it felt, and, panic-stricken, it had begun to fight for its life. It had tried to destroy the womb. For this destructive motion it was punished by being thrust out into the cold and then in having its stomach hurt, 'banged'— which analysis showed to be the pain felt when the umbilical cord was severed. After this first assault on its person it was set aside in a blanket. This covering was uncomfortable and constricted its movements. It imagined that it had been transposed from one womb to another. Because its new womb caused it discomfort it wished to rid itself of it just as it had done the other. For on emergence from the uterus it thought it had succeeded in its efforts in destruction of the womb. It now made another motion in anger. Again the aggressive act was followed by assault, this time from many fingers that inflicted innumerable little hurts. The handling of a new-born child is painful to a skin and the underlying muscles which hitherto have experienced nothing harsher than amniotic fluid. It was bathed and dressed. The cold, the unpleasant tasting water and the being moved and turned first this way and then that, caused acute suffering. To the infant it was all part of the chastisement. Finally, it is bound tightly in a binder which, because of its sore and throbbing cord, was extremely painful. Thus it is again hurt, 'banged', in the stomach for having defecated in anger. (It is impossible here to go extensively into detail, but every item of discomfort and pain during this process was brought up in rapid succession in analysis.) Even then painful experiences were not at an end. It soon discovered that every time it made a motion it was 'attacked' in a similar fashion, that is, made to suffer the discomforts of being cleaned and having its stomach 'banged' anew. The repetition of events made the infant feel, more than ever, that its motion was something that was not liked and that it was essential to restrain this act in the future. Once again energy had to be commandeered from the main flow to be used in withholding the physiological impulse to defecate when the occasion arrived.

Still further details, however, were brought to light. Since the infant could no more control its motions absolutely than it could urination, it had to seek a means of dealing with a situation similar to this. It discovered that it could delay attack, so it thought, if it did not strain. It had sensed that it was when it had strained (accompanied, no doubt, by grunting) that it was attacked (lifted out of its cot for attention to its napkin), and that when it was not straining, that is not getting a 'red and hot face', it was left undisturbed. It argued, therefore, that it was safe to make a stool if it did not 'push it out'.

If it came out of its own accord, without effort, then the infant would not be punished. So energy had to be further controlled. The patient had already realized that hate added to the full strength of an all-out effort increased the effect. It was such an effort that the baby had used to destroy the womb. All-out effort, therefore, had become fused with hate because of the early combination of hate and energy, and so the infant was unaware of its capacity to make a complete motion without hate. It also realized that exertion coupled with hate was the strongest effort it could make. That is, in fact, true. The strength of a homicidal maniac, or a man defending his life, is far greater, as we know, than any consciously deliberate exertion made in an unemotional state. The infant had only known this kind of effort in relation to stool-making. The very first two times it had defecated the act had been allied to a massive fury and hate, due to the imagined necessity of having to defend its life. Thus energy used in a full, forceful motion had become merged, indissolubly, with hate. It found, too, that its fantasies of destruction had the same hate-to-destroy element in them. Since the use of hate-force in the expulsion of its motions did not stop attacks, but rather, so it seemed, brought the attacks upon it, there now existed the need to preserve itself from a recurrence of punishment for its stools by some other way. It was in a dilemma. Especially as by this time it had also found it could not, even if it wished to, completely control its natural evacuations. Its experiences led it to the belief that it was this hate-force, the 'pushing out' with all its might in anger, that was being punished. Therefore it would stop 'pushing' altogether. And when the motion could no longer be withheld it was allowed to come out of its own accord, without 'pushing'. Avoidance of holding its breath and of forcing and grunting succeeded to some degree. It deferred the assault on its person for a time, for the mother, not hearing the usual noises, did not attend to the child till later. When the cleaning up did begin the lapse of time between the evacuation and the appearance of the parent severed the continuity between the act and the result, so the baby did not connect the two events in its mind. Therefore, its device to control attack was felt by it to have been successful in this instance. It had made its first classification with regard to modes of defecation. A forceful stool was dangerous because it would be followed by an immediate onslaught. A gentle stool, unattended by 'pushing', that is force, was safe and was not followed by attack.

Let us now see what effect these early experiences had upon the adult. Throughout life the patient had suffered from chronic constipation, to the degree at times that medical assistance had been needed. He took an undue time over his motions. An evacuation without the least force behind it is not a quick process and, further, a relatively small stool is made this way. The baby had found that, in addition to not 'pushing' and thus having a gentle evacuation, only a little fecal matter came through. Because it was not attacked after this it reasoned that big motions were forbidden and little ones were not. In order to assist stools without 'pushing' and to have them in safety, the patient had always carried a book with him to the lavatory. Reading, it had previously been discovered, symbolized breast-sucking. This precaution had two advantages. The infant had never been attacked while at the breast, for no one had interfered with it there, even if it had made a motion. This assurance of lack of interference meant he would have ample time to make a stool without effort. If he was to hold up his motion and not 'push', he needed time for the peristaltic wave to come, which would of its accord, and without effort on his part, result in a small unforced stool. That kind of motion was the safest the infant could make. The small motion, also, would not make the noise of a large one and so draw attention to it in the cot. And, lastly, the small stool would not smell as strongly as the copious and frequently gas-laden complete stool would do. All these factors came in to make the incomplete stool safer.

Why, we may ask, when time had healed the umbilical cord, did the child not then, on experiencing no further pain attack after stooling, realize that it would not come back? The answer to this query is that it felt it had learned a way of controlling the attack, and that the absence of attack was due to this control. Nor was it likely to risk an acute trauma by experimenting to find out whether it, the pain attack, had permanently disappeared or not. One would not enter a field in which there is a wild bull because one could not see it any longer. Inquiries would first be made as to why it had vanished from view. The baby was not capable of making inquiries.

Its experience had been that it was violently hurt in its stomach by a 'banging' pain if it did a large, all-effort motion. Until analysis could show that that attack could never happen again, its defenses had to remain.

Since this last fragment of material came through into consciousness the analysand has completely lost his constipation. The need to suppress effort in stooling, to protect himself from attack, was at an end.

As in the case of urination, fear in the act of defecation had reverberated in every activity in life. No matter how energy was used it aroused anxiety. This anxiety was built up of fear relating to urination and of fear relating to defecation. Fear of defecation added its particular quota to anxiety in the act of concentration. With relief from fear in both these activities (urination and defecation) a marked change in the patient's power of concentration, in his ability to work for long periods on a task, and in his memory, all of which require forceful and continued effort, immediately followed.

'Tiredness' and 'headache', the signals used as warnings against an approaching onset of a paroxysm of muscular spasm, were also used as indications of impending danger in the anal situation. With the completion of this phase of analysis, the necessity having been removed, both warnings ceased to function. The release from tiredness and headache permitted him to work for as long as he wished or the task required.

His freedom to throw off all restraint was demonstrated soon after the discovery of the meaning of the foregoing unconscious material. He sat down to do some drawing and found himself scribbling. He used his pencil heavily, straining long and hard, as if at stool, grunting and groaning all the while. When this was finished he went to the lavatory and repeated the straining and groaning while he actually made a motion, one which was complete and satisfactory. He noticed, too, that he had no hot and aching head from the straining, which he had usually experienced after any sustained effort.

As a final illustration of the damming-up of energy I will give an incident relating to the function of breathing. The subject had been reviewing the material of his analysis and had sighed with relief as he realized how many unconscious fears of his had been resolved. This had taken place before he had gone to bed. When in bed that night he found himself breathing very heavily and, because of this, unable to sleep. He therefore decided to investigate its cause. At this stage he had almost completed his analysis and was able to carry on the work to some considerable extent by himself, between analytic sessions. His mind immediately connected up with cigarette smoking. While many strands of the causes that forced him to smoking had come up and been cleared, he was by no means yet free of the necessity to smoke. He noticed that he smoked most frequently now when at work. Then followed a careful revewing of the exact manner of his smoking. He became aware that when working he held his breath and that because of this, after a while, he would have to relax. It was then that he would promptly light a cigarette and inhale deeply, breathing heavily while doing so. After several inhalations the cigarette would be snuffed out and work would be continued. Then he wondered why heavy breathing was his way of expressing relief when an unconscious fear had been fully resolved. His mind took up this trail, and the next query was on what other occasions would he, as an infant, need to breathe deeply from relief. It was during breast-feeding that such a necessity would occur. Smoking, then, symbolized the deep breathing as a relaxation at intervals during breastfeeding. It had already been realized that anything gained through analysis constituted a breast-feed. Understanding, or knowledge, symbolized breastfood. Thus, when he had completed a bout of analytic work satisfactorily (that is imbibed milk), cessation from analysis (that is the wthdrawal from the nipple) was a release from the strain of work (that is sucking was followed by the heavy breathing of relief). The deep breathing after a completed bout of analytic work had always been felt by him to be due to release from unconscious strain.

The compulsion to breathe heavily vanished at this point and he turned over to sleep. But now he found himself driven to a change of breathing. He was taking a short breath, which was succeeded by a period of a minute or longer in which he did not breathe, and then another short breath and again a pause. It was a frightening and uncomfortable experience; and since it continued he decided to do more self-analysis. He focussed his attention this time on breastfeeding. When would an infant be compelled to breathe in this fashion? he asked himself. Coördinating sucking with breathing would take some time to install after birth, he thought, and until able to do so the infant would split the functions—sucking when not breathing and breathing when not sucking. Therefore, when the heavy breathing of relief came after analysis it was because he had had a satisfactory suck and could now release the nipple and breathe freely; and the short breaths and long pauses was how the baby first coped with the problem. There was still something as yet unsolved for his mind continued its search. His thoughts then led to the question of what might happen if the infant breathed while sucking. It would choke. That, then, is why it holds its breath while sucking. And the act of work was an equivalent of the act of sucking, for unknowingly he had been in the habit of holding his breath while working.

He felt he was progressing; but all was not yet clear. Immediately another change of breathing occurred, as if in answer to the feeling that something was not yet clear. His nose became blocked and he was forced to breathe through his mouth. This was the indication of how choking came about. While occupied with sucking the baby's nose would have been pressed against the breast, and when needing to breathe again it would have been compelled to do so through the mouth. This it would do while still sucking, and choking would result. Choking was, so the infant would feel, the punishment for sucking and breathing at the same time. This is what must have happened, thought the patient, and to avoid this hurt the baby devised a splitting of the functions. It sucked as long as it could, then released the nipple and took a short deep gasp and then continued sucking again, alternating sucking and breathing in two separate acts.

Cigarette smoking, however, was an improvement upon this, for when he inhaled he sucked and breathed deeply at the same time. A cigarette, for this reason, was the ideal nipple, for he could suck and breathe without choking. When at work anxiety would arise after a period of concentration on his task. He would have to stop. Two or three deep inhalations would relieve him of the anxiety and he could then continue the work. But as we have seen, smoking was serving a double purpose. It not only relieved his held-up breathing, which concentration on his work brought about, but by inhaling the smoke he assured himself that he had a breast handy which did not inflict a choking if he breathed and sucked at the same moment. The cigarette smoke was substitute breast-milk.

All these aspects became clarified the next day when discussing the problem with his analyst. Its effect upon him was instantaneous. For the first time he began masticating his food instead of gulping it down, as had been his custom. He realized that he was breathing while he ate. He had previously been unable to masticate his food long enough as the compulsion to breathe deeply forced him to swallow his food quickly to enable him to do so. He was now able to enjoy the full flavor of his food. His chronic indigestion began to improve from then onward. An explanation of another character trait followed. He had never been able to work at two tasks at the same time. At business, if taken off one job to attend to a more urgent one, he would get angry and distracted. Doing two things at one time was the equivalent of breathing and sucking together. His complaint was that he could not concentrate on both jobs at the same time. Concentration, when the infant was sucking at the nipple, was a necessity in order to remember to hold back breath so long as it was sucking. Interruption in this concentration was disastrous, for it brought about choking. In adulthood his inability to adjust to quick changes limited his capacity for coöperation, not only at business but at home. Any interruption constituted a dangerous interference to concentration, even when he was only occupied with so small a matter as unimportant reading.

The inhibition in breathing had also affected his physical development. He was unable fully to take part in the usual exercises of the young. He was short-winded. He had to hold-in his breath while concentrating on running. Since most activities in waking life require concentration of some sort or another, he became addicted to shallow breathing. There can be little doubt that lack of the full use of his respiratory muscles has contributed to some extent to the development of his pigeon-chest. His body finally had become accustomed to shallow breathing and had established it as a 'natural' rhythm.

Another phenomenon arising out of inhibited breathing was a restriction to his power to show pleasure. It arose in the following way. Beauty was connected, in the unconscious, to breast-feeding. When he saw anything beautiful, such as a landscape, his emotional response was so great that it created a feeling which he likened to choking. The emotion of pleasure made him breathe deeply. To breathe deeply, when in the act of enjoying beauty (breast-feeding) was too dangerous, and so he received a warning—a sensation of choking. To safeguard himself against this feeling when in the presence of beauty the emotion of pleasure was thus unconsciously checked. He could not be exuberant. It has already been shown how this barrier to enjoyment had been increased from other unconscious sources.

As in the case of his other activities, the need to inhibit breathing was but one more example of deflection of energy from the main current. To hold back breath instead of breathing deeply is energy used in a negative way.

It has now been shown how this infant had dealt with five major situations, over each of which it was an urgent necessity that it should gain control. I shall briefly recapitulate.

Firstly, the experience of the muscular paroxysm, which was controlled by suppression of anger. Secondly, the headache, which was controlled by suppression of crying to the point of strain, and avoidance of situations which would bring about crying. Thirdly, the circumcision, which was controlled by inhibiting and regulating the flow of urine. Fourthly, the birth experience, the repetition of which was controlled by inhibiting muscular activity and by anal restrictions. Fifthly, the choking, which was controlled by inhibiting breathing.

In every case the goal aimed at was control. The purpose of control was to escape pain. A large proportion of the infant's energy was diverted from the natural channels to obtain a mastery of its surroundings. Almost the whole of its life was taken up with the struggle to retain control of its environment; and this continuous conflict was reflected in the character of the individual in adulthood. He dominated where he could; and where this was not possible he thwarted authority and thus assumed a negative control of a situation. It was not possible for him to ask for things since this would imply that he was in a subservient position, and to be so would mean he was not in control. For the same reason he could not admit lack of knowledge as this would be to admit inferiority. He talked authoritatively on subjects about which he knew little or nothing and in this way kept himself in a parental position; that is, he assumed the position of authority.

As his analysis progressed his character changed. Each unconscious revelation brought about a tangible result. The need to control his anger having been dissolved, he became normally aggressive. He could ask for things he felt he should have or share, instead of doing without. His domineering attitude disappeared and his need to thwart authority faded away. His aggressiveness had formerly been of a negative character, never direct aggression. This was manifest in his obstinacy, argumentativeness, refusal to accept learning from others and in declining any suggestion made to him. Now, for the first time, he was able to assimilate from the world that surrounded him. He was able to accept suggestions and new ideas instead of instantly refusing them. His breathing became normal while working and he no longer became irritated at interference. Slow mastication of his food occurs at every meal. To enumerate every change that took place would take too long for they entered into every crevice of his mental and physical life.

Incidents and details of the processes of the infant mind relating to the apportionment of its vital energy could be multiplied, but enough has been given to demonstrate the harm that deflection of energy from its normal direction can cause. I shall, therefore, now confine myself to a brief discussion of the following points: (1) Was the infant's method of disposal of its energy satisfactory? (2) Could it have surmounted its difficulties in any other way? (3) Could anything have been done which would have protected the baby from those sufferings?

In the first place we must consider what disposal the infant, as a result of its repressions, made of its energy. As we have seen, its energy had become split into two parts. The main body of energy was used in an inverse way, as a holding-back. It requires a considerable amount of dynamic force to check a body in motion. Reversing the direction of energy means first halting the forward going movement; and then propelling it in another direction. The wastage of energy caused by this is obvious. The analysand had lived life holding back his natural activities. Leg and arm energy, pleasure energy, crying energy, anal and urethral energy and, finally, the energy of deep breathing were all grossly impaired. As a consequence his body is poorly developed. After birth and circumcision, that is after the first fortnight of life, the patient was forced to hold down his cries to the limit of his capacity. We know full well the infant who is a feeble crier, who whimpers when it should be screaming its protests. Such a baby develops poorly. We should expect an ill-development of its chest. The patient of this story is pigeon-chested. Failure to use muscles leads to atrophy and a partial failure to ill-development of the part of the growing organism affected. Thus lack of muscular development can be one of the factors in the malformation of bones. The patient did not walk till quite late and has a slight degree of genu valgum and pes cavus. It might be suggested that this was due to rickets. But inquiry and observance goes to show he was not affected in this way. His pigeon-chest and kyphosis were largely the result of postural errors, and these, in turn, were due to poor muscular development. The endocrines also play a large part in development. The effect of strain and fear on the endocrine secretions is profound. As fear reacts chiefly upon the adrenals, we would expect to see physical evidences of this. At the least excitement the patient would become pallid. I have myself noted such affects frequently. His pulse would become rapid and, on occasions, fluttering.

All through life he has lost the health-giving deep breathing and accelerated blood circulation of full muscular action. His circulation was poor, he was anemic, his skin was dry and he suffered from chronic acne. His bowel-wall, too, would have suffered from the general atonic condition of his muscular system.

Because the major part of his energy was directed in a negative way, he had little free energy with which to meet the every-day necessities of life. The available measure of vitality was still further modified because at the first sign of tiredness he has had instantly to collapse. He has had to function within narrow limits.

What changes should we expect on release of energy in this respect? Here is the answer. Whereas, at one time the patient's power of using muscular energy was so poor that after an hour's physical labor he would be exhausted and pallid, he now can work all day without exhaustion at such heavy work as gardening. Concentration as we have seen requires energy, and expression of energy in this direction was forbidden through its connection with sucking and breathing at the same time. The shallow breathing habit, which fear had imposed upon him, led to lack of the full oxygenation of his tissues. His brain was anemic. This anemia has disappeared. He can now concentrate for hours at a time, throughout the day, on work that demands unusual mental activity. Because memory is a matter of concentration this, too, has vastly improved. Finally, his physical condition has improved in every way. He has developed color and his complexion is no longer muddy. The acne has cleared up and his circulation has improved.

It has been shown, by the case under discussion, how energy can be displaced at its very source and can become a destructive force that affects the physical and mental growth of the individual. It has also been demonstrated how these negative forces have been reflected in his character traits. Further, we have seen how this patient's dynamic vitality had been deflected to meet and avoid attacks, and how the energy at his disposal was used aggressively in a negative way. With such a major displacement of energy from the main stream we should expect to find little free energy left. This was actually the case. In order to use the small amount of free energy left to him, an intricate system had to be built up. He must only employ his strength in a miserly way —a little at a time. He must never attempt to continue exerting himself when tired; and the avoidance of tiredness was arranged for by seeing to it that he had plenty of sleep—far more than an adult usually needs. He used a relatively enormous amount of his free energy in getting to and fro to the cinema, often driving fifty miles or more, on occasions, for that purpose. As long as danger was kept out of his daily life he could be more active. Therefore, he evaded doing anything in which his will was, or might be, thwarted. He read late at night when he should be sleeping, thus again avoiding being thwarted. The bed, which symbolized the womb, was a place where interruption did not come. The use of his eyes had not been attacked so he was free to make use of energy in this direction. As reading was a free channel he used it almost to the extent of actual injury to his eyes. Because there was no unconscious threat in injured eyes this did not deter him. His night reading only stopped when his eyes had become bloodshot and painful. Where channels were open he was avid to use himself to a point of exhaustion in obtaining the allowed pleasures. Exhaustion brought on in this way was not alarming because there was no threat of punishment behind it.

From this summation of ill effects brought about by deflection of energy, in the case of this infant, it is now possible to answer the queries previously set out.

The answer to question (1) is an emphatic No! The disposal made of the infant's energy was not satisfactory. It was most unsatisfactory. Question (2) is also answered by a negative. The baby's experience was insufficient for it to make any other adjustment than those it did. To question (3) the reply is both Yes! and No! Some of its sufferings could have been avoided and others could have been mitigated. Certainly circumcision could have been omitted. In the majority of cases circumcision is in no way necessary; but if performed, whether on medical or religious grounds, the operation should be done under anesthesia. Although birth can in no way be avoided the progress of the fetus through the pelvic canal can, to some extent, be controlled. 'Twilight sleep' may possibly be valuable in respect of easing this part of the birth trauma for the infant. It is a matter for us to find out if this be so. Treatment immediately after birth can always be improved upon. With all these considerations, however, there always must remain some degree of shock at birth and the infant mind will respond instantly to its first experiences of suffering by building up defenses against their recurrence. For the complete and untrammelled use of its potentialities every child should have an analysis at an early age.

In conclusion, I wish to draw attention to one other point relating to the patient. In spite of his character traits and his poor physique he was, to the average person with whom he might meet, a very ordinary and 'normal' young man. No one considered him neurotic. No one appeared to notice his lack of staying power. These deficiencies were all taken for granted. The reason for this, as we know so well, is that we are all, in varying degrees, in a similar situation. Birth traumata have left their mark on each one of us. We have all become inhibited and are driven by the unconscious far beyond the limits of our awareness.

It is only when deep analysis has finally exposed the unconscious deviations of our vital force, from which we have been suffering, that we become aware of what we have lost in the dynamic enjoyment of life.

Note

1 This article was first published in the *Psychoanalytic Review* (1941, 27:305–326).

Chapter 7

Lecture on Surrealism[1]

I chose the title of this lecture so as to leave me free as to what I should say on this subject. Like all new movements of interest, Surrealism is many-sided; and in one short hour it would be impossible fully to cover the subject—nor to treat any one aspect of it in any but the briefest way possible.

I have therefore decided that a short description of its advent into the history of TIME, its development up to the moment of the outbreak of World War II, and the particular contribution that my colleague, R. Mednikoff, and myself have made to it, will cover all the time-space allotted me.

To speak of the birth of Surrealism into the sphere of modern art I must first mention what immediately preceded it, namely, Dadaism.

Dadaism made its appearance during the first world war. A number of artists insensed and maddened by despair at the imbecility of war, and at the various governments responsible for bringing about war, as a council of despair decided to act as they felt all responsible people in power were then acting.

It was a method of meeting the enemy with his own weapon, so they felt. Demonstrating to the world the imbecility of the social organisation, by throwing on to canvas and paper images of madness. By exhibiting behaviour in a like vein.

It was like a skin eruption, in the body of the human: the throwing out from the social body of the toxins that were poisoning its whole system.

It was the outward manifestation of the sickness within.

I do not mean by this that the Dadaists were themselves aware of this taking place. They were only aware they wanted to act themselves as madly as they felt those who governed them were acting.

They did not realise that their own inner psychological stresses were the prime cause of this eruption. We all try to ease our inner disharmonies by projecting them on to the outside world.

Never in history had the outside reality, the actual imbecilities of those governing the world, become so apparent to the oppressed masses that

DOI: 10.4324/9781003333098-7

compose mankind. War always leaves both victors and vanquished in a very much worse condition than before.

The artists—that part of the body politic more sentient and, therefore, quicker to express the inner needs of mankind, succumbed to this eruption of destructive behaviour, for Dadaism was a destructive movement. It was a madness which exploded into the world of art and, after a short duration, as quickly died out.

Out of this explosion of madness Surrealism was born.

During the period of Dadaism the aim was deliberately and consciously to express oneself as crazily and viciously, i.e., hurtingly as possible. The whole public through this was to be aroused to a like craziness.

Exhibitions, fantastic, wild, stupid, revolting and even hurtful to the Victims were shown in Paris, Cologne and elsewhere.

To give you an example, let me describe one which appeared in Paris in 1922—the last Dadaist exhibition. The approach to the exhibition hall was darkened. Meaning and groaning came out of this darkness. The Visitors, especially important ones, were loudly insulted. One artist would meow like a cat, another repeat idiotic sentences ad nauseum, a pair of them shook hands and continued this performance for long periods on end. The artists all appeared wearing white gloves and no ties—and so on. They recited so-called poems. The ABCD poem and the 1234 criticism.

After a short four years the disease which had spread like measles to many art centres in different countries suddenly subsided.

Internecine war began within its ranks and it died, so to speak, overnight.

Amongst the many artists and posts within its ranks were a few who, although discontented with Dadaism, had felt the impact of the bizarre that came to the fore during this period in the so-called art productions. There was a certain quality of beauty to be discovered in the marvellous.

Among these artists and poets were Andre Breton, Soupault, Apollinaire and others. During the reign of Dadaism these few came together and discussed the marvellous creations that sometimes erupted out of the chaotic mess that was being produced and flung at the public. They had discovered that all was not lost—there was something constructive that could emerge from all this.

In 1919 Breton and Soupault practiced automatic writing together and were astounded at their results. This was taking place while Dadaism was in full flood. In 1920 when Dadaism had waned Andre Breton formed a group. Apollinaire coined the word 'Surrealism' during one of their discussions. But it was not until 1924 that Breton defined what Surrealism was. Then he gave the following definition:

> Pure psychic automatism, by which it is intended to express, verbally in writing or by other means, the real process of thoughts. Thought's dictation in the absence of all control exercised by the reason and outside all conscious aesthetic or moral preoccupations.

Surrealist art is not new. The name only is new. The aim of Surrealism is new, but not automatic productions—that is works that are products of the Unconscious.

Before I go further I must explain what is meant by the Unconscious. There are two regions of the mind. One part is conscious and the other unconscious. The unconscious mind contains all our forgotten memories right back to the womb. All experience is registered on the mind. Out of all our experiences we build up ideas, or fantasies, which are from all periods of our existence, from infancy onward. When these appear in consciousness they are irrational, fantastic and sometimes alarming in form. Of such material are dreams made of and we all of us have experienced dreams of every kind—some pleasurable, others macabre and nightmarish. Automatic drawings and writings come from this lost or inaccessible part of the mind and every true automatic drawing or painting or poem is of this character.

As I have already said, Surrealist art is not new. Centuries ago, in Greece, it was a part of every man, woman and child's life. Greek mythology contains some remarkable Surrealist images. There was the Minotaur—half man and half bull: Satyrs—half man and half goat: Centaurs—half man and half horse: Sirens and Harpies—half woman and half bird. The best Surrealist images of all were, first, Scylla, who had six heads on six long, very long, necks, twelve feet and twelve arms: second, the Hydra, which was a nine-headed serpent: last, the head of Medusa whose hair was composed of snakes and who had large glaring eyes which turned men to stone.

Today we are equally at home with Surrealist imagery in the fairy stories we read as children. The finest example of which was Lewis Carroll's story of Alice in Wonderland.

Almost everything about true Surrealist creations seems utterly absurd. And yet, with an understanding of the story behind the irrationality, it will be found that every line, shape, colour and association is deliberately chosen by the psyche because of the symbolic meaning of each object and juxtaposition of objects. Unconscious selection and arrangement is a reasoned process for all the apparent incongruity of result.

True automatic works are hieroglyphic inscriptions of memories buried deep in the unconscious mind, wherein every episode and experience in infancy and childhood is recorded. And every individual has a different system of hieroglyphs.

I have digressed somewhat to give those of you who are unacquainted with psychology an inkling of what is meant when we speak of the unconscious mind. I have also shown you that Surrealist art is as old as the hills.

I will now return to the group who christened themselves Surrealists in 1920.

Andre Breton had, during the second world war, been attached to a psychiatric hospital as an orderly. During this period he had come into touch with many of the manifestations of unconscious creative work of the patients, and with doctors who were using the Freudian method and other methods of bringing the unconscious into touch with the conscious realm of the mind. He also read Freud's works, and so, when he talked of automatic productions, theoretically he knew what he was talking about. But to know about these psychological methods and to practice them are not one and the same thing, as we shall presently see.

Andre Breton then started group action. They experimented together in automatic production, and soon disaster followed. The unrestricted eruption of unconscious behaviour led one man to commit suicide. Breton was not a trained analyst. He was in a similar position to a man who having read a few books sets out to do a dangerous operation. Fortunately he was quick and honest enough to realise this and gave up these group seances. In future each artist or writer worked on his own, and each used his own restrictions. These restrictions are self-imposed by the Unconscious, and therefore acted as a safeguard.

But after a while, proceeding in this way, they began to feel baulked. What they had expected to happen did not happen. There is a psychological reason for this halting of the automatic material coming through which cannot be gone into now.

Andre Breton had stated that the liberation of man would result from the merging of the Unconscious with the conscious. Man could not know what he was and what he wanted until this had happened.

But the liberation of man had come to a standstill, as soon as he abandoned the group seances.

Since the ultimate liberation of man was the drive and aim and force of this movement, that energy had to be turned elsewhere.

He withdrew his eyes from within and now looked outward. If liberation cannot come from within, it must come from outside. But how? Revolution was the answer. The breaking up of the whole social organism. We must smash our way to liberty.

Overnight the movement became revolutionary and had returned back to Dadaism. From this time on Breton published manifestoes periodically declaring that liberation of man could only come by social revolution first. Liberation of man from within was relegated to a back seat.

How it is time to tell you where and how my research work linked up with Surrealism.

In 1935 I had a 'hunch' as a result of working for many years as a psychoanalyst. As a result of this I decided to make a research along the lines of this 'hunch'. At about the same time I met Mr. Mednikoff and in talk with him I realised here was a god—sent opportunity. Would he come in with me in this research. I told him briefly what risks he would run—that both he and I would be the guinea pigs of this research and so on. Anyway, to cut it short, he did come in with me and the results have been more than in my dreams

I had hoped for. The psychological experiment I was making led us into the realm of art; automatic art and writing were frequently in use. And with what success or otherwise you will be able to see to some slight extent this evening.

In 1935 an International Surrealist Art Exhibition was being held in London, England. We had not heard of it and, at that time had no notion what Surrealist art was, nor had we thought then of exhibiting our works at all, etc. (story of our advent into this Exhibition and what followed).

I have with my fellow guinea pig, from working towards the same end as A.B. had laid down in his theories of Surrealism. But only by chance had I worked in this medium, I was researching into the psychology of so-called normal man.

I have given you the briefest history of Surrealism up to the present. I will now say a few words on what we can find in Automatic art and why it is an important form of art, and, lastly, how to enjoy a Surrealist creation.

It is human nature to push off or push away anything new that approaches us for the first time; so I warn you, any of you who may be seeing some of this work for the first time—don't be alarmed at the way you may react.

The unconscious part of one mind will speak to that of another—deep answers deep—and your response will be automatic. It is not necessary for you to understand the painting or drawing as the ease may be—simply look, enjoy if you can, or if you are repulsed, accept that emotional response—don't fight it.

In an exhibition we held in Cork street 1939 in London, one was astonished at the multifarious responses of those who came to see it. For example, one man was particularly enraged at one picture. He spent a long time in the gallery and came back again and again to the one that enraged him. In the end he liked that painting so much he wanted to buy it, only it was not for sale.

His first response was one of fear. After he had recovered from that he was able to absorb from that painting an experience which finally made him want that painting.

Automatic art is important. It tells the tale and expresses for us all the fantasies, and many of them very beautiful fantasies, for which we need outlet.

As art, I will leave others to judge. So far I have found traditional artists and artists of all shades of opinion have come to feel true automatic art has value as art. All artists speak of having a message in their art. Their satisfaction in their creations largely depend upon the degree to which they feel they have put it into their work.

Any artist who has practiced automatic art has found it help him in this respect. The freedom he has found by this practice has been carried into his everyday art, the form of art that is his natural vehicle and choice. I speak from personal knowledge when I say this.

Many artists and poets have come to us and we have initiated them into this form of art expression. Both in London and Cambridge exciting results have occurred. One (...)[2], who was a poet, was thrilled when he found his power of imagery went far beyond anything he had previously experienced.

Surrealism has widened the aesthetic horizon by establishing a new conception of art, that of the value of the 'marvellous' and the beauty of irrational thought and creation, and has courageously made use of the symbol language of the psyche to demonstrate the thesis that emotional life is a major part of the whole personality which, if nurtured and developed, will increase the consciousness of social good. It is true the Surrealists were not aware that the Unconscious was actually 'speaking' through art, but, nevertheless, they knew, as all artists throughout the ages have known, that art was a medium for communicating the thoughts of the inner self. The Surrealists presented to the world a visible manifestation of the creative activity of the unconscious.

Not only is the vitality in a true Surrealist creation greater than will be found in traditional modes of art expression, but the automatic painter develops an individual sense of rhythm, balance, appreciation of pattern and form, and a very personal attitude to the use of colour. The variations are as numerous as the changing cloud shapes that scutter across our skies, as numerous as the population of this world. Such variety is not found in traditional schools of painting, ancient or modern. It could not be so for such works were and are created within the limits imposed by the acceptability of traditional thought and by habit bound public opinion.

I have briefly sketched for you the Surrealist movement—how it arose out of Dadaism and travelled towards a goal—how it met inevitable difficulties and how it split in two—one group going one way and ourselves another—how these two groups are going to the same end by two different routes. By eruptions and revolutions on the one hand, by understanding and reconstruction on the other hand. The work goes on, as it must go on, whether under the flag of Surrealism or revolution or any other flag, for the liberation of man is an emotional urge within each one of us, and one that in the end cannot be denied. As we become more emotionally and creatively conscious we bring the day of our deliverance nearer.

The creative urge is within each one of us, and as I shall show in the publications that will follow this research of mine, is part of a biological rhythm and therefore a biological necessity.

Only to the degree that that creative urge within us is liberated shall we experience individual freedom.

Surrealism, by bravely accepting the true worth of the personal side of creation has helped to establish the belief, which all mankind holds, that fantasy is a legitimate activity that all have a right to enjoy. It is fighting for the encouragement of the personal act of creation for all, as opposed to the right and ability of a few to enjoy this privilege. We are all potential creators, having within us the divine spark that will ignite the creative flame. We are all personally interested in creation, whether we know it or not, And, ultimately, the personal, the automatic, the psychic aspect of creative effort will be recognised as the power behind art. Surrealism is but one of many beginnings of this inevitable trend towards the liberation of man.

Notes

1 This lecture was given at the Vancouver Art Gallery, Canada, on 14th April 1944.
2 The original three words are illegible.

Chapter 8

Surrealism and psychology[1]

Many of my listeners may not have heard of Surrealism before so I will begin by giving you an idea of what it is.

It is a modern form of art which started in France in 1919. It was born out of Dadaism, which immediately preceded it. So first a word on Dadaism.

Dadaism sprang into being during the last war. A number of European artists, incensed end maddened to despair by the imbecility of war, and at the governments responsible for the war, decided, as a council of despair, to act as they felt the people in power were acting. It was a method or meeting the enemy with his own weapon. They demonstrated to the world the imbecility of the social organisation by throwing on to canvas and paper images of madness, and by mad behaviour. It was like a skin eruption in the body of the human – the throwing out from the social body or the toxins that were poisoning the whole system.

I do not mean by this that the Dadaists were themselves aware of what was taking place. They were merely easing themselves of pent-emotions. They were only aware that they wanted to act as insanely as they felt those who governed them were acting. But it was their own inner psychological tension which was the prime cause of this eruption. They were projecting their inner disharmonies on so the outside world.

Dadaism was a destructive movement. It was a madness which lingered for a short while only in the world of art, and then quickly died.

Out of the ashes of Dadaism Surrealism was born.

Because of dissatisfaction with Dadaism. Andre Breton and several others started to experiment with automatic writing in 1919. Andre Breton had worked as an orderly in the psychiatric wards of war hospitals and had become aware of the marvellous creations that some of the soldier patients produced. These, as he had learned from the works of Sigmund Freud, sprung from the unconscious mind. He felt that automatic art should have similar results – that they, too, should be marvellous creations; and that through these the unconscious mind of man could be discovered and

DOI: 10.4324/9781003333098-8

understood. Groping his may thus he finally defined pure psychic automatic work as Surrealism.

Before proceeding further, however, I must explain what is meant by the term 'unconscious mind'. There are two regions of the mind. One part is conscious and the other unconscious. The unconscious mind contains all our forgotten memories right back to the womb. All experience is recorded in the mind. Out of all our experiences we build up ideas or fantasies, which are from all periods of our existence, from infancy onward. When these appear in consciousness they are irrational, fantastic and sometimes alarming in form. of such material are our dreams made. Dreams are varied in content—some are pleasurable, others nightmarish, and more often than not are irrational.

True automatic drawing: and writing: come from thin loot part of the mind and they possess the same characteristics.

Most true Surrealist creations seem utterly absurd. And yet, with an understanding of the story behind the irrationality it will be found that every line, shape, colour and association of objects is deliberately chosen by the unconscious mind. They are selected for their symbolic value, and for the telling of e story.

Automatic creations are hieroglyphic inscriptions of memories buried deep in the unconscious mind. And there are as many different systems of hieroglyphs as there are persons.

You now have, I hope, some idea or what lies behind the phrase 'unconscious mind' and, therefore. know with what automatic art deals.

Andre Breton, after he had formed his group and initiated the Surrealist movement, began group-action. He and his followers experimented together in automatic production. Disaster, alas, soon followed, for the unrestrained eruption of unconscious impulses led to a tragic accident. Breton was not a trained psychoanalyst. He was, to some extent, in the position of a man who, having read a few books on surgery, sets out to perform an operation. Any patient would be lucky to escape damage from such untrained experimentation. Fortunately, Andre Breton was honest enough to realise this and gave up group work. After this each individual worked on his own. The over-stimulation of the unconscious mind by group-action was thus avoided.

Andre Breton now changed the aim of Surrealism and directed his own baffled emotions and that of his followers outward, and from this time onward a political trend wan given Surrealist activities. "If the liberation of mankind cannot come from within," argued Breton, "then it must come from outside." But how? Revolution was the answer: the breaking up of the whole social organism: we must smash our way out to liberty. Overnight the movement became revolutionary and had returned back to the destructive attitude of Dadaism. The liberation of man from within, or, in other words, the scientific approach to the understanding of man's mind, was relegated to a back seat.

Nevertheless, Surrealist art survived, for some of the artists were not interested in the political turn of events. They were only interested in automatic art.

Automatic art is easy enough to do. Every time you take up a pencil and begin scribbling, while waiting at a telephone for a call and your thoughts are not concentrated on what you are scribbling, you are drawing automatically. You are not consciously aware of what your hand is creating. You are not in a trance, but your mind is not consciously interfering with what your hand is making the pencil do. What you do in that way is automatic and very similar to the way a Surrealist drawing or painting is done. The puzzle to most people in how a skilfully finished Surrealist work can be produced automatically without the conscious mind taking part in the production. Freedom from conscious interference, to some degree can be attained through practice in this form of automatic scribbling; but full freedom from conscious interference can only be brought about by a method devised by myself during e research into the psychology or the so-called normal man. This, of course, cannot be elaborated here. Time does not permit. But when such automatic creations are produced, they have certain qualities, which are so vital and forceful, that they inevitably elicit an emotional response in the onlooker, sometimes of pleasure, sometimes disturbing, and, at times, of antagonism which can be quite violent in character.

All is not Surrealist art, however, that is fantastic or bizarre. Much co-called Surrealist art is not automatically done; but is consciously fabricated. For this reason Surrealist art has frequently been brought into disrepute. People sense the artificiality and dislike it.

In the case of true automatic art, here, too, the first impression may be that of displeasure. The shock of the strange newness of the creation may at first displease; but with closer acquaintance, after the effect of the shock has worn off, appreciation begins to develop. Many true automatic creations, even so, are beautiful; even though unusual and surprising in appearance.

During an exhibition of some of my works in London, one visitor was particularly enraged at a certain painting. He spent a long time in the gallery and came back again and again to the picture that enraged him. In the end he liked that painting so much that he wanted to buy it, only it was not for sale. His first response was one of fear. After he had had time to recover from that emotion he was able to absorb from the work an experience which finally made him want to possess the painting.

It is human nature to push away anything not that approaches us for the first time; so I warn any of you, who may be seeing works of this kind for the first time, not to be put off by your immediate reaction.

The unconscious part of one mind will speak, as it were, to that of another—deep answering deep—and the response will be automatic. Further, it is not necessary to understand the meaning of the painting or drawing to enjoy it—simply look. Enjoy it if you can; or. if it repulses you, accept that emotional response—don't fight it. Then go back to the work again and then again.

Surrealism has widened the aesthetic horizon by establishing a new conception of art, namely, that or the value of the marvellous and of the beauty of irrational thought and creation.

It is true the Surrealists were not aware at the beginning that the 'unconscious' was actually 'speaking' through art; but, nevertheless, they knew, as all artists throughout the ages have known, that art was a medium for communicating the thoughts of the inner self. The Surrealists presented to the world a visible manifestation of the creative activity of the 'unconscious'.

Not only is the vitality in a true Surrealist creation greater than that which will usually be found in traditional modes of art expression, but the automatic artist develops also an individual sense of rhythm, balance, appreciation of pattern and form, and a peculiarly personal attitude to the use of colour. The variations are as numerous as the population of this world, for each person is the product of his or her own particular reservoir of experiences. Such variety is not to be found in traditional schools of painting, ancient or modern. It could not be so, for these works are created only within the limits imposed by traditional habit-bound thought.

The work of Surrealism will go on for the liberation of man is an emotional urge within each one of us, and one that in the and cannot be denied. As we become more emotionally and creatively conscious we bring the day of our deliverance nearer.

The creative urea is within each one of us. It is part of a biological rhythm and, therefore, it becomes a biological necessity that it should find full expression. Only to the degree that that creative urge within us is liberated shall we experience individual freedom.

Surrealism, by accepting the true worth of the personal side of creation, has helped in establishing a readiness to accept the fact that fantasy is a universal and legitimate activity that all have a right to enjoy. It is fighting for the establishment or art as a natural means of expression for all, as opposed to the idea that it belongs to a talented few. We are all potential artists, having within us the 'divine' spark that can ignite the creative flame. We all wish to create, whether we know it or not. Ultimately the automatic or unconscious drive behind creative effort will be fully recognised as the power behind art. It is only in so far as an artist is able to express himself completely in his painting that he becomes great. Surrealism is but one of the many indications of the ever-mounting insistence on the liberation of men, for the freeing of mankind can only come through the releasing of the creative spirit within each one of us.

Note

1 This lecture was given as a radio talk for the program 'Mirror for Women' (Canadian Broadcasting Corporation) on 10th July 1944.

Chapter 9

Draft summary of psychorealism

The sluicegate of the emotions[1]

The springboard of thought

The mind begins to function prior to birth, at the point when the foetus is first affected by certain intra-uterine experiences. The birth process and the early events of post-natal life continue this shaping of the way the mind functions. The first significant experience is the beginning of uterine contractions, which according to GWP/RM are a counter-reaction by the muscular walls of the womb to the lively kickings of the foetus in the late stages of pregnancy. Birth is an agony of indescribable tortures for which the infant's rudimentary mind can find no explanation. Pain is its lot from the various handlings it undergoes in its early days, and sleep provides its only relief. It is helpless in the face of all these hurts, but when it finds that certain of its actions are followed by increase of discomfort or pain to itself, it tries to help itself by preventing, or at least restricting, its activity previous to the onset of pain. Thus, an attempt is made to restrict crying, because too much of this causes headache. Evacuation of its bowels leads to being removed from its cot and being subjected to handling of its body while its nappy is being changed. In the GWP/RM terminology, it fears these "attacks" or "punishments" which continue, because after all it has little control over its natural functions. Hereafter, any activity which is not followed by these disturbing procedures represents a lessening of its fear. First comes breastfeeding, which is not followed immediately by an "attack", and this applies also to dreams, which are real to it. But a satisfying and protective dream can also be interrupted so that the infant can be cleaned up and bathed. Just as other events which were followed by "attacks", such as kicking (leading to restriction of movement) and crying (followed by headache) were real enough, so must the wished-for events of its dream, followed too by the discomforts of handling, also be real. To the baby, the acting out of a wish or impulse in dream life is now as real and as dangerous as its other instinctual acts. Now GWP/RM describe how a very complex system of defence-mechanisms is set up allowing the dream to take on a different form, in which guise the apparently disapproved-of wish succeeds in emerging. This development occurs within the first weeks of life

DOI: 10.4324/9781003333098-9

and continues throughout infancy and early childhood and into adult life in a process of stratification, layer upon layer. This limbo of forgotten ideas, desires, memories, fantasies and fears, this storehouse of infantile suffering, the repressed part of the mind, has been named the "unconscious". Although forgotten, it remains active throughout adult life.

The account then goes on to explain the permanence of the division between the conscious and unconscious aspects of the mind. The split arises in the first place *as a defence mechanism* to support the infant's greatest aim, that is, the desire for freedom from pain. The part which is in contact with the outside world has itself two sides, one calm, capable and able to prepare against possibilities beforehand, the other timid and easily liable to lose control over itself. From the former side, a section arises whose sole function is to warn when danger is at hand. The rest of what is left of the efficient side of the ego maintains its directorial and controlling assignments. Under the protection of the two divisions of the personality which remain conscious of the outside world, the timid ego basks in the pleasures of dream existence.

Next, GWP/RM turn to the situation where the infant is increasingly exposed to contact with daily life, e.g. through less hours of sleep, and also the beginnings of an order imposed on it by parental control. Even before it has acquired speech, it has felt the need to convey to its parents the needs which have arisen in relation to waking life. This it has done by symbolic behaviour. When the parents have responded favourably through sensing the general drift of the message, even though the symbolic language has not been understood, the child becomes encouraged to use symbols. The more the parents understand *the exact nature of its wants*, it will be the less likely to suffer needlessly.

The next chapter is devoted to a description of symbol language.

Symbol language

Knowledge of the value of symbols is obtained within the first weeks of life. It grows in the nursling from observing the effect of its behaviour upon the parent, and of once more applying the principle of cause and effect.

When the infant cries it discovers the mother is instantly close by. A crying sound, therefore, is realised to be a means of gaining attention. Because it cries when damp and uncomfortable it assumes that its noise tells the parent of its predicament. Noise symbolises the need for attention.

[From this point, the authors' account is complex and detailed, and to omit even one link in their chain of argument, which would be inevitable in a summary, would not do justice to the chapter as a whole. I prefer, therefore, to reproduce the next two paragraphs in full, in the hope that they will act as a guide to the summary which will follow. D.R.]

Crying is also thought to be a sign of its wish to hurt since it always makes this noise when angered and wanting to hurt whatever is causing it pain, and because it is usually "attacked" after it has expressed itself in this way about the cleaning-up and bathing it so frequently gets. It thinks it is "attacked" for its signs of anger, and the wish to hurt. It is also aware that when it makes such a sound it feels a hurt in its head – from headache. Because it experiences this pain and is also "punished" for crying, it presumes that the infliction of suffering is retaliation for the hurt its noise must have likewise caused the parent. It reasons that if the sound it makes can hurt it (the headache), then it is also able to hurt others. It is convinced that this is the case because of the distress which follows from diaper changing, which it feels as retaliation. Crying or noise is in this way imagined to be a way of hurting others, as well as being an indication that it wishes to attack, or that it has made a mess.

An angry sound is not only a symbol with two meanings, it is also a dangerous activity because it hurts the mother who then retaliates. Because of this it becomes necessary to make some distinctions so as to prevent a recurrence of the painful consequences of hurting with noise. The crying that is intended as a hurt, and that which indicates the need for attention, take on different characters. Screaming with the *full power of the lungs* becomes the indication of the wish to inflict hurt and of actually doing so, for that is always what it wishes to do when forced to shriek with the agony of an acute pain. Such high-pitched noise comes when it is terror-stricken at the feeling of the stomach-binder being unwrapped, for it knows that this is always a prelude to an unbearable hurt, and its shrieks are attempts at hurting the hands busy unbinding it in order to prevent them completing their task. And always this loud, full-throated noise brings on the additional pains, so it feels, caused by the lifting of the navel dressing. Thus, noise made with all the available energy at hand, is dangerous, and is interpreted as an act of destruction and a sign of the wish to annihilate the attacker. Ordinary crying does not bring such results, and it is not instantly followed by pain. Furthermore, a less-piercing noise only comes when a milder hurt, such as hunger or discomfort, is felt, and the mother never fails to interpret such a sound as meaning a need to have these distressing conditions removed.

Crying can be taken as a paradigm for other acts, which also acquire specific meanings, according to the results which follow. Apart from these acts, meanings become attached to the various objects with which the infant comes into contact, such as the breast, the nipple, the nappy and so on. The breast is like a large ball, the nipple like a much smaller one. Not only shape but also colour, movement, texture, light and warmth are further associations adding particular meanings to a symbol. Also, things alike in colour or shape become interchangeable. The infant at the breast gazes into its mother's eyes, and, warm in her arms, sees the twinkling of light in her pupils. These, the source of pleasurable visual sensations, become identified with the nipple at which it is sucking at the time and soon follows the fantasy of eating them. The fantasied eating of the pupils is related to the wish to take in the attractive pleasure-giving orbs, and thus the imagined act is transformed into a reality. [Cf. Ben Jonson's *Drink to me only with thine eyes*. D.R.]

Colours, and even variations in hue, receive specific meanings which vary for each individual child according to the environmental stimuli to which it has been exposed. The text contains a wealth of examples. [Here I give only one, relating to the colour black. This symbolises deep sleep, absence of any awareness of light, dirt, dirt as something not liked and bad, dirt that can hurt. The figure in Plate 8 illustrates this last theme. D.R.]

The application of symbol language in early life

To exemplify this "hieroglyphic system of communication", the authors use the reactions of a child of eighteen months, who still wants to be fed from the breast, though aware that this is no longer allowed, while at the same time a new baby has arrived and is being suckled. Being fed would satisfy his hunger and also lessen the pain of his existence. His mother must really know this, but he has to convey to her exactly what he wants, in spite of his poor resources of speech. [Though the theme is a hackneyed one, the authors' understanding of the infant's thought processes is on original lines – hence I again find it necessary to quote them verbatim.] The child, therefore, begins to act out the story of its needs in play. He knows that he was fed after being cleaned up, when he was the only baby. The breast milk was given after he had given his offering to the mother. A dirty piece of paper is soon found and presented to the parent. It symbolises a dirtied diaper, the "gift" that must precede the feed. The offering of this "gift" is making known his wish to the breast and is indicating his love and desire to be loved in return.

Or else the child might offer the baby a ball, or if that was not available, any article coloured pink or yellow, so that it should not be without a breast equivalent, leaving the mother free to give him the real breast.

If it seems that after all, the mother is more interested in the baby than in him, and that she is quick to attend to it following its continual wetting, the latter would seem a desirable habit. But past experience has told him that he gets scolded. But in the boy's mind, there are links with a time when he could wet without being scolded. He used to be fed at the breast covered with a blue shawl which tickled him, and this excitation caused him to pass water with pleasure. Blue became linked with that kind of situation. If his mother accepted his offer of the "gift" of a blue object and responded either with a feed or with tickling him, it would indicate her permission and wish to have him wet.

Alas! Mother does not understand and in any case has only enough time to take the object in some safe place. The boy will cry and suck at anything available or feed himself in the form of a doll or any object, using any other object as a breast which feeds. If his mother only enters into the play. it gives the child a sense of security in that it is getting attention to its needs and that the fantasy or wish in the play is at least permitted by the mother.

If all these efforts fail, then play will serve as an outlet for the hate that has been aroused, with banging of objects or the tearing of the very object that was offered as a "gift" to induce an equivalent gift from the mother, e.g. a piece of wet paper, denoting a wet nappy. Although the tantrums of an angry child are known to be a reflection of its desire to hurt the parent, it is not realised that its play is acting as substitute for speech. Furthermore. it is not yet thought that the inarticulate infant still unable to walk possesses this symbol language. It is this unawareness that makes the child's life more difficult than it need be.

[It is hardly possible to summarise the authors' micro-dissection of the process of the dissimulation of fantasy and of its pathway to lying without doing it an injustice. Instead, I shall reproduce the last three paragraphs of this chapter for their own measured comments. D.R.]

We have seen that the trend of all activities is towards the achievement of protection from pain and that the mother's love and admiration are thought of as symbolic of her desire to protect those whom she loves from any unpleasantness or suffering, which includes all discomforts, pains, fears and deprivations. Also, that the new-born baby is unable to tell of its sufferings or needs in a manner that can be understood by the parent; and that its only language is the manipulation of symbols, which, in later life, is manifest in the play of the child. By means of this symbol language the infant and child attempt to talk to the parent and select their fantasies or symbolic stories on the basis of their susceptibility to the omnipotent power that rules their world. Those fantasies which are punished or not liked are either hidden under a facade or given a false meaning or purpose.

Lastly, no matter what the conditions of suffering that follow its acts of imagination are, the child continues actively to employ itself in fantasy creation, increases its defences in ratio to the dangers that confront it, and, subsequently, in later childhood finding greater safety for imaginative life in admitted or admired forms of play since by these means concealment is more effective.

It should therefore now be no surprise that in the adult creative activities of mind the infantile or unconscious mind is still actively employed in the pursuit of happiness and freedom from pain, and that the fantasies of gratification are constructed with the aid of symbols of many kinds.

Art as communication, and for gratification

The authors start from the generally followed custom of parents giving their children paper and drawing materials, often with the declared intention of keeping them busy. For the child, however, there is more to it than that. Here the fantasy finds an outlet in a drawing that, especially with the very young child, is almost always greeted with approval, even if the fantasy behind the scribble is one that is not usually permitted.

This theme continues into adult life: adult art is a developed skill in the use of symbols, of shape, line and colour, and still remains the language of the undeveloped, inarticulate and timid side of the ego even while associated with adult ways of life. In support of this view, and to dispel any doubt in the reader's mind that representational art can serve the unconscious in the way indicated, a pencil drawing of a landscape near Piddlehinton, Dorset, is reproduced (Plate I). It was made by RM at a time when he had no knowledge of, or contact with, psychology or its adepts, and several weeks before he joined GWP in the research, of which this book is one of the fruits. He had been attracted to the scene by the presence of a village pump and a gnarled tree close to it.

The subsequent analysis of the content of the drawing centres around these two features, which then appear as symbols of his mother's body, which in his fantasy as a young child he had damaged because she had denied him the food he wanted, and of her breasts which, like the old village pump, didn't give of their liquid food – a throwback to the time when he was two and still occasionally wanted the breast but was refused it because it was all going to the new baby.

The authors do not always reconcile the two aspects of the child's graphic efforts, namely, its need to hide its secret fantasies, in which its demands upon its mother contain a destructive, therefore forbidden and punishable element, and on the other hand, the importance of making known to the parent as clearly as possible what it wants. But it appears that the child gets to understand that the more skilled the work is, the greater will be the parent's approval, which, once more, means love and security and freedom from fear. Only in this latter sense can the subjection of the child's mode of drawing first to the parent's ideas of what is correct, and subsequently to the standards of the parent-substitute, the art-teacher, have value. At the same time, forbidden aspects of the fantasy involved can still remain hidden.

Although art is, perhaps, the most suitable agency for the safe expression of unconscious desires, it does not necessarily follow that it is the only medium with this advantage. Its superiority over other known methods of approach to the psyche lies in the fact that it is, at present, the only way by which a documentation of inner thoughts and fantasies can be made. By means of its use a record of the feelings and processes of the infant mind, from before birth and onwards, can be obtained in factual form.

Such records have been compiled. They have provided the material which has made possible this narration of the development of an infant's mind. Because the value of art as a vehicle for unconscious expression was recognised before the research began, much of the investigation was carried out with the aid of colour, shape and line. As a result of this, there is a wide choice of material from which to select representative illustrations to demonstrate various phases of mental behaviour, as well as to prove the worth of art as a psychic outlet with unlimited scope.

The destructive impulse

This chapter describes the induction of the child into the code of behaviour expected of him within his first society, the family. Not only are there so many things that he must do or that he must not do, but it seems that the decisions of the parents are often arbitrary and directed against him, for the very things that are allowed on some occasions are denied at others. The authors contrast the outlets available for the adult to work off his anger from frustration in energetic physical activity or verbal aggression with the limited means available to the child, especially when very young. As it becomes aware that even these means, such as screaming or kicking only result in further restriction, its hate and anger become channelled into fantasies of destruction directed against the author of the controls. Even these fantasies have to be shut away from awareness, in the first place from others, but also from itself, because they are dangerous. The authors thought that there was as yet neither widespread understanding of the causes of aggression nor recognition of the need for its release. The only method that could be of social value would have to be a preventive measure that could be administered to very young people during the early period of formal education.

In the meantime, the research carried out by the authors had led to the evolving of a way of partially alleviating the strain resulting from the inhibition of aggressive impulses. The way was through art – through a particular kind of automatic art. This was not merely a physical way of releasing pent-up emotions. It was necessary to disable or destroy the enemy, for it was this action that dissipated fear, which, in turn, dispelled the need for aggression. Art, with its employment of symbols, was the means of achieving both a release of tension *and the direction of this energy* at a symbol representing this source of danger.

The social orientation of the authors is shown in the following passage: An ever-present problem confronting us is how to assure ourselves and coming generations from a repetition of the terrible world catastrophes that periodically arise. It must be apparent that the imperative needs should be to restore equilibrium to war-shattered minds (of the children in particular), to psychologically re-educate youth whose minds have been distorted to ways of hate, and to revise all systems of education in order to permit and encourage the controlled deflation of the unavoidable infantile aggressive impulses.

The destructive impulse revealed through the language of symbols

Most of this chapter is taken up by the interpretation of symbolic language as exemplified in several drawings and paintings, all done according to the principles of automatic art, the exact nature of which is explained in the following chapter. Photographs of the original works are available, but the minutely detailed interpretations, which in any case are not readily assimilable, would be quite meaningless if summarised. I present here, therefore, the interpretation of just one watercolour painting (Plate 2), and the introductory paragraphs of the chapter.

How, where and when the destructive impulse is in action will now be demonstrated by a selection of a particular kind of automatic work. These will reveal unconscious infantile feelings in various situations. Whenever possible corroborative conduct in our common daily life will be given. They will also illustrate the destructive impulse in action in relation to the various people with whom a child has to live; but these illustrated episodes are not *final models* of the nature of these activities since such patterns are varied in each individual. The infantile situation giving rise to the destructive act illustrated will also be presented.

It cannot be sufficiently stressed that the destructive urge is not the only type of impulse that obtains egress by this method. Emphasis is here laid upon this impulse because of the way it influences our everyday responses to whatever impinges upon us during the carrying-out of daily tasks; and because it is the most frequently used of the defences evolved by the infantile unconscious.

Within the limits of this revelation of the psyche much will be learned of art itself. In realistic or representational art, the choice of colour is logical and restricted by the usual appearance of the object being painted. In automatic art, colouring is not bound by rules or rational associations. A horse may possess a yellow ear, a pink eye and a blue and green coat. Everything about such creations may seem utterly absurd. And yet, with an understanding of the story behind such irrationality, it will be found that every line, shape, colour, object and association is deliberately chosen by the psyche because of the symbolic meaning of these things, and of the juxtaposition of them. Unconscious selection and arrangement is a reasoned process for all the apparent incongruity of result.

These works are hieroglyphic inscriptions of memories buried deep in the unconscious mind, wherein every episode and experience in infancy and childhood is recorded. They cannot be erased. In the research carried out by the authors, by long and persevering effort this language was deciphered, and it was discovered that every individual has a different set of hieroglyphics.

The examples presented here are drawn from the material collected during this research, and were translated in every detail, but only those parts of the interpretations will be given here that are relevant to the topic under consideration.

The first story is of a little girl. The incident to be narrated occurred when she was eighteen months to two years of age. Her brother, elder by eleven months, persistently interfered with her game. He was at an age when he wanted to possess whatever he saw was providing pleasure for the younger child. She was never free from his depredations and too weak to fight him off. And it was always the most cherished of her toys that were taken from her. Whenever she gave vent to her rage, the nurse, who displayed a marked preference for the boy, punished her instead of her brother. To add to her difficulties, the little girl was unable to talk well enough to be able to disprove the brother's lying explanations to the nurse. The need to find a reason for the brother's interference and the nurse's punishment led her to believe that they did not want her to have the fantasies that were incorporated in her games with the toys. The brother's interference was his way, she thought, of obstructing her fantasy, and the nurse's slaps were punishment for *wanting* to have a fantasy.

During such a game the baby girl lost a blue ball which was the utmost importance to the carrying-out of her fantasy. It represented a breast. The brother had taken it from her. Her feeling of rage at him dare not openly be expressed for nurse would punish her for displaying her hate of the brother.

This information came through interpretation of a number of drawings and paintings. This tale of the thwarting of fantasy life was an introduction to the action which was portrayed in the drawings that had then followed. In these, an attack on the brother, which previously had been safe to express openly, takes place. The first part of this attack is illustrated in Plate 2.

Here the brother is the large figure with an angry-looking eye. He is being bitten on the leg by a dog, which is a symbol of the baby girl when she is being naughty. To attack the brother is naughty since nurse punishes her for so doing. A dog has been used to symbolise the naughty side of her because such an animal, in an early childhood episode in actual life, had killed a chicken, and in this way was seen to be a creature that could hurt effectively with its teeth. The identification of herself with a dog is in order to be able, in this fantasy, effectively to attack the brother, with the maximum effect. The angry girl in the drawing is herself. It is seen that she can only attack in an ineffectual way by spitting. That is why the wish to be like a dog arises. The creature on the boy's shoulder, which is trying to choke him, represents the baby girl and her wish to hurt the brother in a way which she has learned from experience is very painful. The large claw that swings over towards his eye depicts the desire to destroy that part of him which sees her treasured objects and makes him want to take them from her. The reason why the brother has been drawn with his hands in his pockets is to prevent them being used to attack back, that is, to guarantee herself safety from his hurting hands, and of freedom to assail him.

The unconscious purpose of this painting is to reveal the wish to hurt the brother, and the ways in which she would like to do so, as well as actually to attack him in this manner in painting this picture.

The attack is continued in intensified form in Plates 2 and 3, for each of which there is an interpretation which similarly encompasses every detail of the artwork to such a degree that any summary is bound to lack internal consistency. With this internal consistency, the interpretation may appear fantastic but it does have its own logic. Without it, the interpretation is likely to seem contrived.

The characters in the next fragment of childhood drama is a baby boy of nine months who *in fantasy* has taken something belonging to his sister, who is a little over two years old. Plate 5 illustrates the boy's method of destroying his sister who, out of jealousy, takes every opportunity to hurt it; while Plate 6 shows the details of her revenge. Plate 7 also has as its subject the ferocity of the ex-baby towards the new baby. The theme of sibling rivalry has been well worked over, but these analyses claim to show the links in the chain of argument which leads to the particular fantasied action, and often a novel insight is provided. For example: Thus before the artist [of Plate 7] was able consciously to realise it [the shapeless mass in the fierce creature's mouth] was the baby being killed by biting, the thought was in mind that the dirty morsel being bitten by the creature was being destroyed because it was dirty. It was being destroyed because mother liked dirty things [to be] treated so. She does not like dirty things. This the excuse held ready should the mother discover what is really taking place. It is the reason given her for getting rid of the object that is really the baby. In addition, in the child's eyes, father is just another baby who can command mother's love, attention and the food she has to give ... He is as great an obstacle to the child in its attempts to obtain the mother's unstinted love – the love that is felt to be an assurance of absolute safety from harm. There follows a socio-political extension of this theme, not easy to summarise, in which Hitler and the Nazis are equated with the older child and the Jews with the helpless baby.

The drawing reproduced in Plate 8 illustrates an attack upon a father figure. This is one of the drawings which were used in GWP's (1938–39) article "The scientific aspect of surrealism" (see Chapter 4 in this book). There, GWP summarised its content as follows: "This drawing of a man having his eye gouged out has in it the wish to get into the father to find a safe place from an unsafe external world. The reason for the need for flight is also stated in this picture. The man's tongue is torn by his own teeth, in disapproval of himself. The drawing is expressing fear of the man who would do such a thing to himself as punishment for his own misdoings, and "If," it is argued, "this is what he does to himself for his bad behaviour, what would he do to me if he caught me wanting to behave badly? I must find a good way to escape his anger". And so a hole is bored into the man and a hideout is found in his body. The act portrayed by the infantile unconscious, about which this fear had arisen, was that of stealing milk from the mother". This summary takes up close on 200 words. In the work being here summarised, the interpretation of the drawing and accompanying comments, including one on the psychological harm that can result from too early religious training, occupy nearly 2000 words.

Plate 9 portrays the destruction of the mother who prohibits the pleasure of eating things picked up from the floor. The detailed analysis is followed by an explanation of the special importance which the artist attached, in producing the work, to making it one that would earn general approval, while at the same time he was not conscious of its significance. In short, the beauty of the work was to disguise its destructive meaning. Equally, beautiful words, like beautiful pictures, serve to transform a repugnant act into one that will meet with approval. History is cluttered with many such instances of infantile cunning.

Psychorealism

The research, for which the claim is made that it reaches further back into the development of the mind of the infant than ever before, now is extended to wider aims, as shown in the following quotation: The pattern of human conduct and thought is established at birth, and it is only by a full knowledge of the way in which the infant develops its fundamental psychological pattern of life that we shall find the means of bringing into balance the mechanism that lack of understanding set awry. And then, when this knowledge is at hand, we shall be confronted with the task of formulating the therapeutic measures proper to the situations to be dealt with. Automatic art is a projection of psychic reality since, in portraying the earliest fantasies of infantile life, it portrays what is real to the infant, a reality which is preserved and extended into adult life, though not in a form readily accessible to the adult. For this reason, the researchers coined a special term, Psychorealism, for their approach. Psychorealism and psychorealist art are automatic creativeness that is *entirely free from conscious interference and selection*. They are the unhindered projection of psychic realities. These results are, at the moment, only obtainable through the method devised by GWP and RM.

The material for the present book was gathered in the years from 1935 onwards, but had its first writing-up in book form when the couple were in the USA, i.e. from 1940 onwards, during the Second World War. They now turn to considering certain psychological aspects of the world situation. With war raging, the psychological solution, even though at hand, is useless while hate virtually fills every crevice of man's mind. It was now not a matter of whys and wherefores. It has once again become necessary in some parts of the world to encourage hate of horrible oppression so that annihilation of the oppressors be speedily brought about. However, the important task is the mental rehabilitation of those children whose minds have been evilly warped and who have suffered indescribable mental and physical torment. In other words, they were then advocating the equivalent of a later "Save the Children" campaign. Psychology had been perversely used in the interests of war and evil – it now had to be used by world leaders for the purpose of good. But in the meantime, psychorealism is offered both as a temporary measure and as the means that will help quash the cyclic events that follow wars and lead to further conflict.

Just as adults could benefit from venting resentments or unbearable emotions in socially permitted ways, so could a child come to realise that it can ease itself from burdensome feelings through psychorealist drawing and painting. It should, from the start, be helped to understand that it is being encouraged to practise this special drawing and painting just because it can do no harm to anybody or anything, and it will quickly grasp the purpose of this special "game". In fact, when the work is an expression of a strong feeling, such as rage, the child will get relief from the very force it exerts in pressing heavily on the pencil or chalk. Physical expression, the expenditure of energy, increases the therapeutic value of such release. The interpretation of Plate 10, representing a violent attack upon the mother, adds a note by the artist: "I dug into the paper as hard as I could". The point is made that in the original situation, the child held back its anger because of the feared terrible parental retaliation. In its place, the child in its sleep would have had a destructive fantasy, which would not have satisfied because of the absence of actual physical exertion. In the drawing, the heavy pressure of the pen upon paper helped to make it possible. The artist experienced much relief from emotional tension soon after this work was done.

Even where the drawing does not obviously depict aggressive activity, as Plate 10 does, and the artist neither had any idea of its meaning while drawing it, nor any feeling of inner stress before beginning it, unlike the creator of the previous drawing – even so, the energy that goes into the making of such a drawing, benefits its creator in almost as satisfactory way as occurred in the previous example. Plate 11 seems to be at first sight a comical caricature, but the analysis of its minute details gives rise to an interpretation of a concealed death wish against his mother, while the drawing itself is structured around a memory of the artist dating back to when he was three years old. In an inconspicuous part of the drawing, his dead mother in the shape of a tiny dead bird, is shown in an equally tiny coffin, and when the artist wanted to name the drawing, the thought "Come back soon" occurred to him, and he gave it this title. Like the drawing in Plate 8, it was reproduced in the article by GWP mentioned above.

The authors now devote considerable space to a descripture of the procedure to be adopted in starting young children on the psychorealist "game". They clearly feel that any self-restraint on the part of the child in embarking on the "game" is due to a fear of revealing its fantasy life, though the child itself might not realise this. Hence the importance of lavish praise, especially in the early stages. Guidance as to the presentation of the procedure both in the home and in schools is given.

Individual and collective benefits of psychorealism

The authors adopt a medical model in discussing the ills of society, e.g., the organisms that ravage the social body are those millions of humans who so easily are stimulated to acts of aggression, The next step is an investigation of the behaviour of the "bacteria". Recent experiments had shown that it was possible, or might be possible, to alter the toxic nature of certain bacteria, in some cases even making them harmless. By suitable methods, including conditioning, alterations could be effected in the organisms that wrack the social body. Why we were unable to examine the deeper causes of our pattern of behaviour was because we lacked the suitable instruments. Just as the microscope came along to enlarge our scope of vision, so psychoanalysis opened up new vistas of the mind. But even Freud's instrument was not enough.

Now, however, psychorealism and the technique of interpreting unconscious hieroglyphs advances psychological science to the stage where an enquiry into the unknown causes of social disorder can be finally completed, for with this psychorealist instrument every determinant and facet of human conduct can be clearly seen, examined and analysed. Because of public indifference and meagre financial assistance, many important findings cannot be published. A complete record of this research has been kept, running into thousands of drawings and paintings, apart from interpretive notes, photographs and other miscellaneous material, but the cost of reproduction, both in colour and in black and white, is beyond what a publisher would care to speculate, particularly as scientific works are not generally "best-sellers".

Amongst the benefits resulting from new psychological knowledge will be a decrease in delinquency and therefore less money spent on prisons and reform systems and their staff. The same would apply to institutions for the insane. Only homes for incurable insanity and for those whose condition was due to physical causes would remain. Of course, money must be found to maintain armed forces to ensure the continued impotence of the one-time aggressor nations and to deter future aggressors. But a small fraction of this outlay spent on the propagation of this new instrument for undermining hate and infusing a new spirit of understanding into humans would ensure the wasteful spending of life and money would never happen again.

Psychologists and educators must collaborate even more closely than before. All teachers must be educated in the ways of unconscious behaviour and trained to apply this understanding of the psyche to the teaching of the young. All willing parents must be given the opportunity of this same psychological training, and centres for psychological information for parents-to-be must be set up. The education of parents and teachers must include the technique of psychorealist expression as a means of deflating the aggressive tendencies in children. Nurses and others who have care of the young must be given training of the same kind. Paediatrists and general practitioners must also be equipped with this new psychological understanding of the young.

Within three or four generations, after the proper functioning of such a system, there will be a greater assurance of peace than by waging useless wars that do not uproot the real causes of jealousy between nations.

The application of the psychorealist method to adults must be in the hands of experienced medical and psychologist personnel. The release of aggressive impulses cannot be given as free a rein as with children. But the very fact that the physical activity involved in the artwork brings with it an element of conscious control, allows for a more gradual emergence of aggressive feelings, while at the same time, pleasure in the progressive unfolding of the creative impulse, probably hidden since early childhood, encourages the artist to persevere. Remarkably enough, the example to be given gets support from a passage in a book by a prominent American anthropologist, Ashley Montagu (1971), *Touching: The human significance of the skin*.

The researchers start from the premise that creativeness is part of the biological or life rhythm, indestructible and unalterable. A fantasy created by the infant may be so real to it, that where it contains a forbidden act, terror of the consequences results, so that the creative impulse has to take a devious route towards less-offending fantasies. Even in play, the handling of objects about the home necessary for the dramatisation of a fantasy may be forbidden, the child not realising that this is done for its own safety.

The hunger to live to one's fullest capacity remains, throughout life, as a dominant need, and that satisfaction is only possible through the fullest expression of the creative instinct; and this is as difficult to satisfy in adulthood, when financial and other circumstances too often frustrate or limit occasions for complete fulfilment of this basic need.

But however restricted the opportunities for creation, the human will strive to create, that is, will still endeavour to compensate for the thwarting in life, and to enjoy fantasy-real gratifications of inner needs. Even in day-dreams, in our "flights of fancy", we are creating, giving form to our desires. But this enchanting practice does not satisfy. It lacks that which conjures up the satisfying sensation of reality, the performance of a physical act which brings the feeling of purposeful endeavour. It is the association of real activity with a fantasy which satisfies the psyche's hunger. It is this that explains why an infant, when dreaming of suckling at the breast, will work with mouth and fingers, sucking and twitching, while asleep.

The remark made by an artist about a psychorealist drawing of his own will bring out more clearly the value of action combined with fantasy.

The drawing he had done revealed the infantile wish to be fed from the breast so as to get the titillation that always came after a feed – the gentle, pleasurable rubbing and powdering after being cleaned and before being put into the cot for sleep.

An outline of a breast had appeared in the drawing at the moment the artist consciously became aware of this infantile wish. With regard to this indication of the mother's breast, he said:

> I suddenly wanted to draw as naturalistically as I was able. I wanted to *make* it real, to use my hands to mould its shape into the real thing.

> Since I was not modelling, I had to use my pen to satisfy this wish and painstakingly shaded the breast *to make it look as real as possible*. I was attempting to make my wish fantasy (of being fed from the breast) into a reality: to bring the actual, the real, the naturalistic breast before me.

The reason for this need for a reality was then disclosed as being due to the unconscious belief that if he could make a real breast from which to feed, the real sensation of pleasurable titillation would certainly follow and, therefore, the full satisfaction of his desire would take place. It was an attempt to transform fantasy into reality. It should be added that this desire resulted from the infant's awareness of the fact that *it was only when he had been fed from the real breast that he was thus gratified*, and that no such pleasurable sensation followed a fantasy breastfeed.

The employment of hands, to experience the making or moulding of an image, was thus clearly shown to be the infantile means of creating a sensation of actuality. The physical act of touching was necessary. In this instance the tactual experience of the breast, which is one of the infant's normal experiences while feeding. was being reactivated in the act of drawing a breast. The stroking movement of the pen on paper symbolised the touching of the breast by the infant. The closer the approximation to reality that the drawing obtained the greater became the *consciousness* of reality; and consciousness of really was experienced by the infant through the sense of touch. Therefore, to be actively engaged with the fingers in drawing a real breast was akin to fingering the real breast, which the infant did while feeding. If the real breast can be created and touched, then the real titillation would follow.

Doing, making or touching, combined with fantasy activity, enables the unconscious to feel it is gratifying its wishes through creative work.

It would be easy to find these ideas attractive, while at the same time feeling that they would have no place in a more objective study.

Hence, it is all the more interesting to read the section on "Touch and painting" in the above-named book, which deals with its subject from a broad range of aspects, supported by references to many sources of information, and I think it worthwhile quoting from the section.

> In the 1895 Bernard Berenson, improving upon a notion of Goethe's that a work of art must be "life-enhancing", suggested that one way of achieving this is by the artist making us imagine that we are enjoying genuine physical feelings when we look at a painting or sculpture. Such feelings Berenson called *ideated sensations*. Ideated sensations exist only in the imagination and are produced by the work of art by making us realise its being and live its life. The most important of the ideated sensations Berenson called tactile values. The work of genuine art stimulates our ideated sensations of touch, and such stimulation is life-enhancing … "Through all the ages", writes Berensen, "and in every place, whenever a

visual representation is recognised as a work of art and not as a mere artefact, no matter how elaborate, smart, and startling, it has tactile values. It may have much more besides, which is more or less of importance or none at all, but to be accepted as a work of art these other attractions must rest on a basis of tactile values, or be in close connection with them". The artist, in creating a work of art – unconsciously for the most part, sometimes consciously – imagines all the sensations felt or which he supposes to be felt by whatever he is attempting to organize and harmonize into an equivalent of what he feels it to be intrinsically, and what at the same time it says and means to us.

The value of acquiring artistic skill is next stressed. The line of reasoning is as follows. The infant learns to distinguish between dream pleasures and real pleasures, and to realise that its pleasure is greater when it is actually powdered than when it dreams it is being so treated. Naturally it prefers the real thing, but, when failing to obtain this, tries to discover *ways of increasing the reality sensation of its fantasies*. The acquisition and application of skill achieve this effect. Much emphasis is placed on the theme that the creative faculty is a part of the system of inter-related biological rhythms, which had not yet been realised, resulting in much mental anguish. Machinery, labour conditions and social conditions have constrained the creative activity of man to a point wherein such expression is curtailed to a dangerous limit. Is it any wonder that, since the psyche's needs have little opportunity for satisfactory fantasy gratification and emotional stress kept at an overburdened point, individuals rebel against conventions, social injustices. industrial tyranny and slavery and, finally, when they can restrain themselves no longer, express themselves in revolutionary activities? The authors see in the will of the imaginative faculty to survive the reason why art has endured through the world's periodic "dark ages". They do not intend to convey through their particular presentation of art that henceforth it should be considered as a cure for all mental ailments. But they do firmly believe that it is an imperative necessity, an essential tool, in the forging of human happiness, and one that has been too long and dangerously neglected.

The creative impulse

Having shown earlier how the destructive impulse functions as a major defence in all situations, real or imagined, that spell danger or the frustration of essential needs, the authors turn to a happier side, the constructive or creative impulse. Because it is a biological need, the psyche continually seeks opportunities for creative expression. even against the impositions of the external world. Since both hate and joy need energy and movement for expression, interference to liberty of action is interpreted by the unconscious as a penalising and thwarting of the expression of hate as well as of the expression of joy. Thus, the belief that the enforced confinement of criminals and the imposition of compulsory tasks. as punishment for crimes committed, will alter character is basically unsound. The restriction to freedom of movement, or even the thought that such freedom is limited, is one of the reasons why those who have suffered prison life bear a grudge against society. Hate of those enforcing this condition upon him must inevitably increase with every hour of his confinement. Socially undesirable behaviour can never be cured by any method employing restrictions to liberty.

The infant's energy is always employed in trying to alter the length and the distribution of the states of pleasure and pain and to weigh the balance heaviest on the side of pleasure. Where it cannot fight the conditions that bring discomfort and pain, its energy is diverted to the creation in fantasy of the desired conditions. This it can do in dream life. Before, it could only try to alter its body position to create physically conditions that would give it ease, now its mind begins functioning creatively for a like purpose.

Most adults are able to exercise their fantasy sufficiently freely to function without fear but within confines set by being trained to behave only in acceptable ways. A good proportion can enjoy fantasy life only by proxy: through the creative works of others, by reading, viewing or listening. But by the time a child arrives at the age it can express itself without too much interference, its personality is already moulded to the pattern designed by its environment, parents and society.

However, there is a hidden fantasy which stirs a child to tear a doll apart to find out what makes its eyes move or the youngster who takes a watch to pieces to find out how it works. They are really interested in discovering how to make a moving, living baby of their own in order to present it to the mother who likes living babies and so to obtain her admiration and love. The chemist, mining engineer, surgeon and bacteriologist all have been attracted to their chosen profession by some facet of the unconscious wish to discover, examine, understand and tabulate the factors that comprise and make the world the thing it is (the world being symbolically the supreme parent figures). What they discover is their gift to the world, which in return gives them admiration. The same social permission for otherwise forbidden activities is found in the arts. In sculpture, for example, the common infantile desire to manipulate and shape what it has produced out of its own body is translated into the shaping of images of beauty from clay or stone.

In the past, art served religion in depicting the stories of the gospel, thus bringing home its message to even the least literate. Since then, art has taken on another function of ministering to the soul in this workaday life. The psyche now can easily find escape, even though temporary, from the miseries inherent in present-day living in the enjoyment of pictures, reproduced or real, in homes and galleries, in listening to music, in watching opera or ballet or films. The developments of this industrial age have led to the spreading of the doctrine that beauty is a necessary factor in good and satisfying living. However, that these are valuable assets to mankind underestimated and hardly recognised as such because they bring neither economic nor practical advantages. Yet, the authors insist: with the increasing complexities of present-day living, art has become more than merely an escape. It is now as necessary as our daily bread and water ... Humanity owes a greater debt to humanity than it knows.

And now art can serve in yet another way, but this time as a revitalising force and in conjunction with science – through psychorealism. Psychorealism widens the aesthetic horizon by establishing a new understanding and conception of art, namely, the value and beauty of the symbol value of the psyche, and, in addition, the use of this symbol language to demonstrate the thesis that emotional life is a major part of the whole personality which if nurtured and developed, will increase the consciousness of and desire for social good. It can also scientifically demonstrate what all artists, throughout the ages, have known; that is, that art is a medium for communicating the thoughts of the inner self.

But merely to demonstrate these facts is not enough. A constructive application of this new way of awakening and re-educating the psyche must be set in action; must be planned to benefit all, or as many as possible. It is in this matter that science can join forces with art. The research, of which this book is an outcome, scientifically investigated every facet of this ancient creative way of transmitting unconscious thought until complete understanding was obtained. The result of this is the formulation of a technique of encouraging psychorealist expression. It offers a safe and scientifically verified procedure for the education in the use of an outlet for emotional tension, under the supervision of specially trained personnel.

Creative fantasy

This chapter uses three works, two in colour and one in black and white, to illustrate the positive functioning of the creative urge, once a position of safety has been reached by the destruction in fantasy of the persons or situations that spell danger. At such times, the symbolic fulfilment of pleasure wishes, the constructive endeavour of the unconscious, leads to creations that radiate the enjoyment experienced by the psyche. Such works are invariably well-balanced compositions; their design, colour and rhythm are dynamic and pleasing; and it has been found that the irrationality displayed in such works is not annoying to the eyes of people unaccustomed to their style. They always impart an unmistakable feeling of having been enjoyed. Each of the works is analysed and interpreted in respect of its details, without reproducing, which it is impossible to form an unbiased estimate of the authors' argument. It is, however, interesting to note that at the end of the argument, they lead on to more general observations wherein they explain a well-known fact by drawing on the analysis they have just made. Thus, they conclude their analysis of the first painting as follows: And so, as if by magic, the fantasy transforms a helpless condition often leading to pain, and the agony and frustration and of being discarded for a new baby, into an experience of transcendental bliss. They continue: The circumstances creating the need for fantasy gratification can partly explain why some artists create their finest works when suffering unbearable conditions. It is possible that in such cases it is only when a state of deprivation reaches a certain pitch of intensity that the creative faculty can become fully active; and then begin to construct the necessary antidote to misery – happiness, the fantasy gratification of all needs. This being the case, a state of want is the best incentive to creation. On the other hand, when admiration is accorded the works of an artist, he or she is encouraged, by this symbolic permission for fantasy gratification, to continue to create similar works. It explains, to some extent, why some artists, having experienced success, develop their abilities to an outstanding degree. But there is another side to this picture of success. When it is easily attained and reaches beyond the individual's capacity for absorption, it leads to a lessening of the ability to create works equal to the artist's best standards. It is possible to explain this phenomenon by the fact that success diminishes the necessity for creating those peculiarly vital works which were essential, before success came, in overcoming unconscious fears of deprivation and frustration. Success brings with it the symbolic gratification of inner needs and so the dangerous situation, which impels the creative faculty to function to its full capacity, no longer exists. Such artists seldom continue painting for long with their initial high degree of vitality once renown and sufficient and permanent financial security is obtained, unless, as in a few instances, other unconscious factors exist to keep the need for admiration at high saturation, even with success.

The chapter ends with paragraphs of glorification of the true purpose of education which is served if all the faculties are developed so that every factor of the body and mind shall function fully and in harmony. Education at present seems to be the development of the individual to a stage of proficiency that will enable him to act and think only to the extent necessary in obtaining the minimum comforts and requirements to maintain a dull life.

Psychorealism, the artist and the "impersonal" in art

The question of the distribution of energy is discussed, of obstructed energy, of energy release, and the value of psychorealism in achieving a better balance is stressed. Psychorealist expression, under trained guidance, serves as a safety valve for aggressive energies, lessens emotional tension, and brings about a feeling for imaginative endeavour. It will not radically cure an individual's mental ills. Its value is that of preventive medicine, helping to check, and maintaining a check upon the harmful consequences of early thwarting and misunderstanding. In this sense it is therapy.

Psychorealism also helps in the development of the aesthetic sensibilities and, if combined with the practical art training, will enlarge a person's potential value as an artist or craftsman. Not only is the vitality of a work increased but the creative worker develops an *individual* sense of rhythm, balance, pattern and form, and a highly personal use of colour. Because we all experience different situations and build up different interpretations of the causes of events, in our infancy and childhood, there are as many variations in the manifestations of our emotions, when such are freely expressed through the medium of psychorealist art. This variety is not present in the works of the traditional, representational schools of painting. It cannot be so, for such works are created within the limits imposed by public opinion and inner fears.

No work of art can be truly impersonal since it is the work of man, of a personality, and calls forth responses from other personalities. A personal element must enter into it because every shape, colour and rhythm has personal meaning and assumes a personal value. This is true even of abstract art because "the selection and arrangement of colours and shapes is essentially the result of the combined activity of conscious and unconscious mind". The universality of great works of art must derive from their "power to satisfy or give pleasure to a central emotional core in humanity which never changes and which, in some way, is alike in all generations – past, present and future". This core is the human preference for all degrees of pleasure end the hatred of discomfort and pain. After a discussion, the conclusion is reached that a work of art possessing "universal" appeal of a lasting quality is one which elevates the onlooker by its presentation of a pleasurable fantasy, enhanced by colour, rhythm and form (which heighten the pleasurable emotions to a satisfying degree); also, that the whole work is able to communicate or stimulate such satisfying, pleasurable emotions in the onlooker.

The main point is that we are all potential creators, having within us the same spark which will ignite the creative flame, and, as a consequence, we are all *personally* interested in the creative, whether we know it or not. Ultimately this utterly personal aspect of creative effort will be recognised as the true spirit behind art and the basis of "universality" in art.

The way ahead

Note

1 This essay has never been published. There is no evidence when Pailthorpe first started writing this paper but she was still working on it when she passed away.

References

Montagu, A. (1971). *Touching: the human significance of the skin*. Columbia University Press.

Berenson, B. (1895). *The Venetian painters of the Renaissance*. GP Putnam's Sons.

Afterword by Desy Safán-Gerard

As read in Montanaro and Stefana's book, Grace Pailthorpe is the first artist and psychoanalyst to have written about how free creative work emerges from the artist's unconscious. She worked as a physician and was an active contributor to medical practice in hospitals and prisons before she wrote about creativity and her experiences while painting. The book describes Pailthorpe's outstanding and progressive career outlining important changes in aspects of medicine and medical care before her involvement in psychoanalytic training. With Mednikoff, her artist/partner of many years, she applied psychoanalytic notions to understand the unconscious meaning of the imagery in her own paintings. Their joint approach and lectures offered in various museums, along with their exhibits, was somewhat linked to the Surrealist movement, when artists tried to translate into their artwork the imagery emerging from their unconscious as it appeared in their dreams and daydreams. Her psychoanalytic training allowed her to write quite cogently about the role of unconscious feelings and phantasies in the creation of new work. She contributed greatly to the appreciation of psychoanalytic ideas by practicing artists, their teachers, and the general museum viewers interested in her paintings.

Pailthorpe wrote papers on the birth trauma, illustrated with her own paintings. Her writings have a close relationship with Melanie Klein's theories. Moreover, she seems to have wished to visually illustrate Klein's notions. Even though she didn't write about the authenticity of the artist's creations, she seems to have given much importance to the artists' acceptance of themselves, however conflicted, and in how their conflicts might be revealed in their creations. But psychoanalyst Brenman Pick, when writing some years later about the authenticity of the psychoanalytic encounter, has questioned how much authenticity we, analysts, and patients, want and can tolerate.

Back to Montanaro and Stefana's book and to Pailthorpe's assertions regarding the legitimate portrayals of her unconscious in her paintings, we wonder, along with Brenman Pick, how much creativity goes into creative inauthenticity. Because, as Brenman Pick (2018) reminds us in her book, *Authenticity in the Psychoanalytic Encounter*, when faced with anxiety we analysts

DOI: 10.4324/9781003333098-10

may be unable to distinguish what is false and what is authentic. Perhaps the authenticity of Pailthorpe's messages from her unconscious that she tried to reveal in her paintings was, in hindsight, only partial. As Brenman Pick has observed, "For even at best we are part authentic and part inauthentic" (p. 132). Though she is referring to psychoanalysts, this also applies quite well to the authenticity of an artist's creations. Psychoanalyst Martin Nass interviewed well-known American composers about their sources of inspiration and concluded that some composers don't seem to be "auditory people" because they don't seem to draw from other musician's work, but from visual experiences, dreams, bodily feelings, thinking feelings, etc. (Nass, 2007). Gifted American composer Bruce Adolphe (2019) has written, eloquently and movingly, about musical imagination and the authenticity in composers at work. He argues, "It is important to keep mystery in its place. Technique, craft, skill – these are not mysterious. But there is mystery in the connecting of craft to feeling, of intellect to intuition, of reason to passion – and that is the secret of creativity" (p. 402).

Perhaps the impressive scope of Pailthorpe's descriptions (found in "Lecture on drawings" in chapter two) could be appreciated in the following notes on the colour symbolism in one of her watercolours: "Here I, the pink object on the left, am definitely and safely ensconced within the womb (blue). The dark surround, which is rhythmical and vibrating, is comforting because of its darkness. The pink body and head of myself is undifferentiated except for one feature: the mouth." This bit of description gives a taste of the close attention to every aspect of her free painting and her subsequent attempts to discover their meaning. For example, she writes: "I wish the placenta-breast that fed me through my belly while inside mother would now feed me, inside mother, through my mouth" (which was the only feature depicted in her painting). I have not come across any of Pailthorpe's contemporary surrealist artists engaging in such descriptions. Aside from being a gifted and committed artist, she was so clearly a psychoanalyst/artist attempting to educate viewers into the beauty of psychoanalysis and its power to explain the unconscious source of the creative impulse. Her generosity of spirit goes hand and hand with her dual gifts as a noted artist and skilful psychoanalyst.

It is inevitable that as a painter and psychoanalyst I would engage in comparisons about what Grace Pailthorpe was doing when using psychoanalytic notions to explain her paintings. Years later I have done something similar while trying to understand and explain my work. However, a striking contrast is immediately apparent: Pailthorpe was using psychoanalysis and especially Kleinian theory to illustrate the elements in her abstract and surrealistic paintings, while I was exclusively interested in the creative process. In this sense, we need to grant her credit for extending to art exhibition viewers psychoanalytic ideas that could be used to understand the creative process. I would hope that the psychoanalytic community was duly grateful to her for familiarising the art-loving public with the importance and value of psychoanalysis to our understanding of the mind and especially their appreciation of the unconscious mind at work during the creative process.

My use of psychoanalytic notions to the understanding of creativity at work is quite different than that of Pailthorpe. I can find examples where I used titles "The Kiss" or "The Fight" to address the content of some early paintings, however I have never been interested in the content of my abstract paintings but very and exclusively interested in the process. I believe this is because some of the creative impulse and the creative solutions emerge from the artwork itself and particularly how artists USE elements in the work or in their chaotic unconscious as a trigger to pursue the work further. Mistakes during the work have a way to energize the artist to search for new avenues and new solutions.

Chapter fifteen in my book *Chaos and Control* (Safán-Gerard, 2018), offers instances where mistakes led me to search for new solutions to a painting in progress, new solutions that enriched and improved the work. For the artist at work, mistakes can be a key engine that moves the work forward in unexpected ways. And there is nothing as exciting for an artist than a new solution to a work in progress. If not an artist, you probably would not share the excitement that a creative solution offers to an artist at work. Art exhibitions are the rare opportunity for an artist to share in this excitement. But can this excitement be truly shared? The Artist Statement, a common practice where the artist tries to explain the work being exhibited, is a bit of an artist's nightmare because it is so difficult to accurately capture in words what the work is about. An attempt for an artist to assert "I am the one who created this!" And to use verbal language for something that is not verbal at all. The audience would not be better off by skipping the Artist Statement and by talking to the artist himself or herself because it would probably lead both artist and viewer to a similar frustrating conversation.

Grace Pailthorpe's brave attempts were based on sound psychoanalytic theory and her experience as an analytic patient to no other than Melanie Klein herself, but I am afraid her lectures about it may have left her audiences confused as to the value of psychoanalysis to help an artist create. What I am saying here or trying to, is that, unfortunately, across such a long time, Grace and I have been trying the impossible: a translation of an emotional, nonverbal experience into something verbal but meaningless to an audience trying to learn about creativity. If that was the case for Pailthorpe, it may have been a sad ending to such brilliant efforts to educate audiences about the beauty of psychoanalysis and its power to help an artist create.

As analysts, we still pursue the truth of our inner experience. As artists, we are only interested in its beauty but only when its depiction is truthful. And how are we artists to pursue and later depict in a painting or a sonata or a symphony the truth of our inner reality? That is the unusual role an analyst can play when helping a struggling or confused artist into allowing that inner truth to emerge, a truth that may need celebrating.

A challenge for both analyst and artist/patient is to allow him to recognise that inner truth, even when wrapped in chaotic feelings that the artist must wade through. The question for us analysts is how difficult it is to become a witness of an artist patient's distress, as he or she pursues a new awareness of himself or herself. How can the analyst help an artist/patient face and use the elements in that internal chaos, as scientists have begun to do with external chaos, into something that can be used in new work? Does the analyst have the strength to help the artist face and tolerate the anguish when encountering disturbing inner feelings? Does the analyst recognise their value as a source of an upcoming creative work? Having gone through creative experiences of his own, the analyst who is also an artist can help the artist/patient USE his new insight. Because such an analyst recognises that distressing chaos and confusion can become useful sources. This involves, of course, a new approach for the analyst where conflicts and chaotic feelings are not to be "resolved" but "USED" as the richest gifts they can become.

In our efforts to understand creativity and to share our discoveries with our artists/patients and with interested psychoanalysts I could point out another difference. Pailthorpe did not attempt to advance her ideas by using a group as an alternative to individual work. My long-standing interest in group phenomena and early training in Gestalt therapy led me to work with a group of artist/patients years ago. Many of my ideas about creativity have been the result of what I learned from my artist/patients discussing their creativity and its difficulties in such a group. I am about to start a new version of a group about creativity that I have called "Expanding the Limits". This time it will not be held in my Venice, California, studio, but will be held virtually.

I have been honoured to have been enlisted with a special assignment from the International Psychoanalytic Association to be the chair of a group of analyst/artists and those who have written about creativity from all over the world. We had our first group meeting during the London IPA Congress in July of 2019. Our most recent meeting was held virtually during the Vancouver IPA Congress in 2021. Despite the distance and language barriers, I continue to learn from our open discussions where members talk about their work with artist/patients and their own creative work. Unusual friendships between members across the globe are a delight many of us share. Pailthorpe would have been a much-celebrated member of this group and its more deserving leader. Her courage to disclose the meaning of the various elements in her paintings in conjunction with the psychoanalytic theory that could explain them will always make her courageous life stand out as a real pioneer of what all of us artist/analysts are trying to learn.

Desy Safán-Gerard, PhD.
Training and Supervising Analyst,
Psychoanalytic Center of California
www.desy.com

References

Adolphe, B. (2019). The Musical Imagination. In: Nalbantian, S. & Matthews, P. M. (Eds.), *Secrets of creativity: What neuroscience, the arts, and our minds reveal*. Oxford University Press.

Brenman Pick, I. (2018). *Authenticity in the psychoanalytic encounter*. Routledge.

Nass, M. L. (2007). The mind of the composer. *American Psychoanalyst*, 41: 18–22.

Safán-Gerard, D. (2018). *Chaos and control: A psychoanalytic perspective on unfolding creative minds*. Routledge.

Index

For Product Safety Concerns and Information please contact our EU representative GPSR@taylorandfrancis.com Taylor & Francis Verlag GmbH, Kaufingerstraße 24, 80331 München, Germany